Advance Praise for *Facing Violence:*

Rory Miller pulls no punches telling the truth in this one of a kind, well written, and compelling guide to survival during and after a life or death encounter. His book, *Facing Violence* should be compulsory reading for all instructors before addressing 'the threat,' when dealing with the criminal mind and body. For those of us that think we know it all, this will be a game changer by helping students understand the truth about the mental, emotional, physical, and possible financial effects of being a victim.

> **Al Dacascos**, martial arts instructor

Rory Miller hasn't only seen the elephant, he's faced it head on and learned from his encounters. He writes about violence and self-defense with the brutal honesty that only comes from someone who has seen the blood, guts, and aftermath first hand. Anyone studying self-defense should take note of the areas Miller addresses in this book. They are critical components of self-defense training. For those of us who teach self-defense, Miller has provided a valuable resource to assist when teaching these principles to our students. And if you aren't teaching these areas in your self-defense classes, you better start. If you are serious about understanding the realities of violence and self-defense, I highly recommend this book.

> **Alain Burrese**, J.D., former U.S. Army 2nd Infantry Division Scout Sniper School instructor • Author of *Hard-Won Wisdom From the School of Hard Knocks*, and the DVDs *Hapkido Hoshinsul, Streetfighting Essentials, Hapkido Cane,* and the *Lock On: Joint Lock Essentials* series

As part of our teaching adults serious martial arts for self-protection, we regularly stress the importance of preparedness—e.g. be prepared to face this, that, or anything else–even the unexpected. A lot of what is 'unexpected' was very well covered in Sgt. Miller's *Meditations on Violence* (critical reading for anyone studying martial arts for self-protection). However, there remains an area of 'unexpected' consequences from which many–even those well prepared for self-protection—are completely unprepared.

Namely, the subsequent police investigations and judicial processes through which the defender must be sufficiently prepared to walk. Miller's new book, *Facing Violence* reasonably extends the defender's preparation to what may very well happen following the successful use of force to protect you, your family, and friends.

> **Bob Orlando**, martial arts instructor, author

Facing Violence **is Rory's gift** to those who would willingly 'step through the looking glass,' as he describes it, to explore interpersonal violence. *Facing Violence* provides the reader with a hint about Rory's style when it comes to getting across his point: direct, intriguing, and often elegant. He wants to teach you seven things about violence, and they're big things. Important things. But the details are important, too—pay attention to them! Don't waste time rummaging around for a lot of 'how to,' look for his explanations of the 'why,' the 'when,' and the 'who.' Look for his treatment of 'capacity' versus 'capability' and his personal riff on 'chaos theory' as it pertains to surviving physical combat, among many, many other nuggets. When you're done reading, read it again. All of it.

Facing Violence isn't a 'fun' read. It's not what I'd term 'entertaining,' in the literal sense. It *is* important and interesting, and will be quite useful to those who've embraced the possibility that violence will touch their lives, and have chosen to prepare.

Lieutenant Jon Lupo, New York State Police, Albany, N.Y.

Assistant Detail Commander of the state police's Executive Services Detail—Capital • Certified New York State Police and the New York State Division of Criminal Justice Services as a police instructor • Certified as a Law Enforcement Instructor in Krav Maga

"The society that separates its scholars from its warriors will have its thinking done by cowards, and its fighting done by fools."—Thucydides

Fortunately for our society Rory Miller is both a warrior and a scholar. Rory is one of those rare men who has encountered violence, survived, and has returned to teach us its lessons. There are many skilled instructors who can make you better at their system. Rory is one of very few who teaches concepts that will make you better at your system, no matter what that system is, and apply that system to violence as it happens in the world (outside the Dojo). *Facing Violence* is a must read for anyone who teaches others to deal with violence and takes personal responsibility for their students to be able survive those encounters physically, mentally, emotionally, and legally.

Officer Kasey Keckeisen, Team Leader/Training Coordinator Ramsey County SWAT • Minnesota State Director One-On-One Control Tactics • Midwest Regional Director Edo Machi Kata Taiho Jutsu • 5th Degree Black Belt Jujutsu, 3rd Degree Black Belt Traditional Kodokan Judo, 3rd Degree Black Belt Yoshinkan Aikido, Dojo-Cho Keishoukan Dojo

Sgt. Rory Miller's first book *Meditations on Violence—A Comparison of Martial Arts Training & Real World Violence* (2008) earned extraordinary praise from seasoned luminaries and 'rookies' whose work takes them into the 'universe of violence.' Truth is, people like underdogs. Who would wager that one of the most consequential books on the world of violence would be written by a career correctional officer? *Meditations on Violence* destroyed the comfortable notion that 25 years of martial arts training make you an expert in real world combat or that being a putative expert in one aspect of violence makes you an expert in all types of violence.

Miller's new book *Facing Violence* is destined to become a classic in the literature on understanding violence. Miller challenges readers to focus undivided and sustained attention to subdue the 'devils in the details' that emerge before, during and after any violent incident. In this authoritative, psychologically sophisticated, and comprehensive text Miller strips us of dangerous illusions and blind spots we have about violence through a careful examination of the seven fundamental elements of violence.

Facing Violence demands that we accept that we will always be beginners in the field we'll call the 'universe of violence.' Miller destroys the foolish and deadly notion that any of us can claim to be an expert on violence. He emphasizes a critical need for humility, fearless self-examination, compassion, and daily practice of the seven fundamentals of violence, for all whose work requires entry into the vast 'universe of violence.' This book is a must read for corrections officers, police officers, security professionals, military personnel, and others who find themselves in martial situations.

Rory Miller is the proverbial underdog who has emerged from the shadows to become an authoritative, distinctive, compelling, and brutally honest voice about life in the universe of violence.

> **Dr. Kevin Keough,** clinical-police psychologist, Doctorate in clinical psychology Baylor University 1998 • Founder of the Marriage and Family Center of Delaware • Originator of North Star Guardians and Warrior Traditions audio interview series • Martial Artist with training in Chinese animal forms, tai chi, chin na, martial qigong, Wing Chun, Tae Kwon Do, and Vee-Jitsu • Author of Music, Meditation, and the Martial Arts of Everyday Life

Miller has enough experience to fill a hundred volumes yet manages to cut to the heart of the matter in one extraordinary tome. His unique ability to make highly complex subject matter engaging and useful makes this a book that every serious martial artist should not only own, but also refer back to again and again. In it you'll discover that self-defense isn't just about fighting. In fact, if your training does not encompass all seven of his principles it is dangerously incomplete.

> **Lawrence Kane**
>
> Author of *Surviving Armed Assaults* and *Martial Arts Instruction*; co-author of *The Way of Kata, The Way to Black Belt,* and *The Little Black Book of Violence.*

When it comes to self-defense, there are Seven Deadly Ignorances. Subjects related to violence that will get you killed or thrown into prison. Rory Miller has cut through the hype and misinformation presented as self-defense training to give you what you need to keep from becoming a statistic.

Miller has taken a massively complex and confusing subject and reduced it to simple to understand, straight forward—and best of all—life saving information.

If you're interested in not ending up dead, crippled, or visiting the prison showers, you need to read this book.

> **Marc Animal MacYoung,** 'nuff said

Once again, Miller has caught lightning in a bottle. Building on the ideas in *Meditations on Violence,* Miller has produced a work that should not just be on the reading lists for our police and military academies, but really needs to become part of their syllabi. It's that good, and I wish it had been part of my training. The core lesson in *Facing Violence* is that fortune, meaning survival, favors the prepared mind. Simple enough. But Miller shows that effective preparation can't be limited to the dojo or the range. In order to be truly prepared, we need to think through moral, ethical and legal issues that are rarely part of self-defense or defensive tactics training. And they need to be. This is a nutritionally dense book and I started my second reading as soon as I finished the first.

> **Robert Crowley,** attorney and former Major, United States Army Special Forces

Sgt. Rory Miller is a philosophical cartographer who spends much of his time mapping out complex ideas on paper. In his latest book *Facing Violence*, his bold and earnest descriptions of the world of self-defense account for the rugged terrain and the natural barriers to living a safe and secure life within a historically violent society. In doing so he represents an accurate social landscape for others to intellectually navigate. Miller has the unique ability to recognize that certain places do exist, and have long existed even though most may deny them being there. Some of the places he takes his readers to are exciting and interesting to explore, while others are frightening locations that most will avoid at all cost.

But regardless, his description of the roadways that lead there is accurate and his gift for preparing both the careless adventurer and the lost navigator a safe way out is compelling. Miller's martial arts and corrections background have helped shape his complex three-dimensional model of survival from which others may vicariously learn. While some may declare that the world of violence is flat, he effectively argues that no, it is indeed round and *Facing Violence* is yet his latest journey into the uncharted legal, intellectual and emotional realms that give substance to his proposed theory.

> **Roy Bedard**, Police officer (Tallahassee P.D.), law enforcement consultant and trainer, former Team USA (Karate), President of RRB Systems International

You need this book. Not just if you are a cop, soldier, martial artist, bouncer, or working security, but if there is any chance you might someday find yourself in harm's way. Miller knows this subject, and if you don't, you need to—what is in these pages can save your life.

> **Steve Perry**, New York Times Bestselling Co-Author of Tom Clancy's Net Force series

Rory Miller is a voice that needs to be heard by anyone involved in real-world violence, be it professionally or in training. This book works perfectly in tandem with his first Meditations on Violence, but stands on its own as well. Rory puts some very serious and confusing information into a form readily understood by both the veteran and the novice.

Pay close attention to this book; too many concentrate on the physical aspects of self-defense/fighting. Rory covers this, but more importantly, he delves into the mind and internal workings needed to survive real world violence. His depth of experience and ability to get it across put Rory's books on the must read list for my students, and that is a short list.

This book will deliver good, usable information every time you read it.

> **Terry Trahan**, Guru; Applied Self Defense Silat/Instructor MSCD Self Defense Course • Former bouncer, event security, knife designer, street rat, survivor

This is quite possibly the most comprehensive book on self-defense training that I've ever read. Over the years I've seen huge gaps in what is marketed as self-defense training, and this book addresses virtually every single one of them. Rory's assessment of the legalities, ethics, dynamics and aftermath associated with violence are the exact things that every responsible self-defense instructor should be teaching to his or her students. This book should be mandatory reading for every serious martial artist.

> **Tim Bown,** FAST Defense (Scenario-Based Training) Certified Instructor & Bulletman • Head Instructor, Safeguard Martial Arts

Sgt. Rory Miller does it again. Following on his seminal book *Meditations on Violence* we can now dive deeper into the critical elements surrounding violent confrontations.

If you are serious about learning how to survive modern day violence, this book will provide you with the definitive guide of the things you need to know about how violent confrontations actually occur and what to do about it.

> **Toby Cowern,** Former Royal Marine • Military Security/ Counter-Terrorism Specialist • Arctic Survival Expert • International Wilderness/Urban Survival Instructor • Operational Safety Specialist • Risk Management Advisor • Firearms Instructor • CQB Instructor

The majority of *Facing Violence* is divided into tutorial units discussing specific elements of violence in self-protection and how they relate to the individual's chaotic aftermath.

In a way *Facing Violence* tells a story. It's a story of liberation, of taking the first steps towards understanding the foundations of emotional survival, beyond the physical.

> **Van Canna,** Uechi Ryu 9th Dan

FACING VIOLENCE
PREPARING FOR
THE UNEXPECTED

FACING VIOLENCE PREPARING FOR THE UNEXPECTED

Ethically • Emotionally • Physically
(. . . and without going to prison.)

Rory Miller

YMAA Publication Center
Wolfeboro, N.H., USA

YMAA Publication Center, Inc.
PO Box 480
Wolfeboro, NH 03894
1-800-669-8892 • www.ymaa.com • info@ymaa.com

Paperback edition	Epub ebook edition	PDF ebook edition
978-1-59439-213-9	978-1-59439-237-5	978-1-59439-236-8
1-59439-213-7	1-59439-237-4	1-59439-236-6

10 9 8 7 6 5

Publisher's Cataloging in Publication

Miller, Rory.

Facing violence : preparing for the unexpected: ethically,
emotionally, physically (... and without going to prison) / Rory Miller.
-- Boston, Mass. : YMAA Publication Center, c2011.

p. ; cm.

ISBN: 13-digit: 978-1-59439-213-9 ; 10-digit: 1-59439-213-7
Includes bibliographical references and index.

1. Self-defense--Handbooks, manuals, etc. 2. Self-defense--
Psychological aspects. 3. Violence--Psychological aspects.
4. Martial arts--Handbooks, manuals, etc. 5. Martial arts--
Psychological aspects. 6. Fighting (Psychology) I. Title.

GV1111 .M55 2011   2011926917
613.6/6--dc22   1105

Printed in Canada

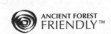

CONTENTS

ACKNOWLEDGEMENTS

Like any book, any exploration of part of the human condition, *Facing Violence* didn't just pop out of my head complete. There have been many teachers on the way and lots of help with the process.

Some of my best teachers have been criminals. The world isn't fair, nor is it balanced in a way that humans understand. The crimes were sometimes horrible, the lessons sometimes invaluable.

Marc MacYoung has become one of my favorite Subject Matter Experts (SMEs). Long phone calls or sitting on the deck, bouncing ideas off the furry little guy is a privilege. He makes me think and often shows me things that I missed. Thanks, Marc.

Paul McRedmond (Mac) has been instrumental in teaching me to see. When I was looking at principles, he was always looking one step deeper. He's always demanded one notch more commitment, one step more depth.

Geoff senior gave good advice when I needed it.

Steve and C.S. Cole, Mark Jones, and K encouraged me to set an impossible deadline for getting this book written. With good friends, impossible isn't that hard.

Alain Burrese kindly offered to vet the legal sections to make sure I wasn't blowing smoke out my ass.

Sifu Kevin Jackson, Rick Prowett, Kamila Miller, and Orion Storm kindly posed with this balding old man for the pictures under the direction of my lovely and talented Kami.

Karen Barr Grossman and David Ripianzi are hereby thanked for the thankless task of herding this from manuscript into something like a book.

Last and most important: This book is for Kami, who has the awesome responsibility of always keeping me sane. *Ti mam rada.*

FOREWORD

There are a lot of books out there on deadly martial arts techniques and killer secrets of the ninja and the ancient principles of various lost fighting arts (I should know—I own most of them). But there aren't nearly enough books on the reality of violence: the precursors, the aftermath, and everything that happens in between. *Facing Violence* is about the reality.

I've been playing around with martial arts since I was a teenager: wrestling in high school, a black belt in judo from the Kodokan, a smattering of karate, boxing, and Brazilian Jiu-Jitsu. And I had some excellent training when I was with the CIA, too. All these systems turned out to be useful—sometimes extremely useful—when it came to the main event. But none of them prepared me for the often ambiguous lead-in to violence (like woofing), or the disorienting affects of adrenaline (like auditory exclusion and tunnel vision), or the shakes and legal complications that come after. Some of these I learned the hard way; others I feel lucky to have learned from reality-based writers like Alain Burrese, Lawrence Kane, Marc MacYoung, Peyton Quinn, and others—and now, from Rory Miller.

If you're in search of a treatise on technique, this probably isn't your book. If you want to study an ancient Asian fighting art, you'll probably want to look elsewhere. But if you want to protect yourself from violence by understanding it better—recognizing causes and signs, knowing how to de-escalate, having a plan for what to do if de-escalation fails, being prepared for the legal and other consequences that can come after—then *Facing Violence* is the book for you. It's smart, it's thoughtful, and it's even funny and philosophical. Above all, it's useful. And a damn good bargain, too, considering what Rory paid in acquiring the experience to write it.

Barry Eisler
Author of the bestselling *John Rain book series*

INTRODUCTION

While teaching a Kurdish lieutenant in Iraq close-combat hand-gun skills, he suddenly threw up his hands and said something. He sounded angry. I turned to my translator and raised an eyebrow.

My translator reported, "He said, 'I am so angry. Everything they taught us was wrong.'"

It wasn't true. He had been well trained on an American model—the same skills that a rookie officer in the states would have coming out of the academy. The skills weren't wrong, but they were incomplete.

Learning to shoot safely is not the same as learning to shoot quickly. Target acquisition on clear firing lanes in good lighting standing upright in a stable stance is very different from target acquisition when holding your head up for a second could mean you eat a bullet. The Lieutenant needed all of the basic skills he had learned. He was just now ready to step out of kindergarten and learn how those skills applied in the world.

Most self-defense training, and especially martial arts adapted for self-defense, suffers from the same problem. Most of what is taught is not *wrong*, but it is incomplete.

There are seven elements that must be addressed to bring self-defense training to something approaching complete. Any training that dismisses any of these areas leaves the student vulnerable:

- Legal and ethical implications. These are different but related factors. A student learning self-defense *must* learn force law. Otherwise it is possible to *train to go to prison*. A self-defense response where you wind up behind bars for years is not a very good win. Side by side with the legal rules, every student must explore his or her own ethical limitations. Some people simply cannot bring themselves to kill, maim or blind. A few cannot hurt another human being. Most do not really know where this ethical line is within themselves. Part of an instructor's duty will be to find that line and either train with respect to it or help the student grow past it.

- Violence dynamics. Self-defense must teach how attacks happen. Knife defense is worthless unless it centers on how knives are actually used by predators. Students must be able to recognize an attack before it happens and know what kind they are facing. The attitudes and words that might defuse a Monkey Dance will encourage a predator assault and vice versa.

- Avoidance. Students need to learn and practice *not* fighting: Escape and Evasion, verbal de-escalation and also, pure not-be-there avoidance.

- Counter-ambush. If the student doesn't see the precursors or can't successfully avoid the encounter, he or she will need a handful of actions trained to reflex level for the sudden violent attack.

- Breaking the freeze. Freezing is almost universal in a sudden attack. Students must learn to recognize a freeze and break out of one.

- The fight itself. Most martial arts and self-defense instructors concentrate their time right here. What is taught just needs to be in line with how violence happens in the world.

- The aftermath. There are potential legal, psychological, and medical effects of engaging in violence no matter how justified. Advanced preparation is critical.

What follows is an introduction to each of these seven areas. Considering thousands of volumes have been written on fighting and each of the other six subjects is at least as complicated—more than an introduction of each of these seven areas won't fit in a single book. However, scratching the surface will show you the uniquely interwoven nature of each aspect and may urge you toward better preparation should your next fight have no rules.

CHAPTER 1: LEGAL AND ETHICAL

The ambulance didn't even leave as a code three. The man was obviously dying and there was nothing they could do. For about forty-five minutes, the time it took for the team to assemble, gear up, and make a plan, the man had been driving his own head into a concrete wall.

We used a Taser to immobilize him long enough to handcuff him. We knew that either the Taser had saved him or we had been too late to save him. We rushed him to the ambulance waiting outside the perimeter. His eyes were being pushed down by the swelling in his brain. His hands and feet were turning inward and pointing down.

While we waited at the hospital, we knew that the very intervention that gave him a shot at living could end in a wrongful death lawsuit against us. Another "Taser-induced killing" despite the trauma the man had done to himself, despite the fact that only the Taser allowed us to get close to him without inflicting more trauma. This was shaping up to be something for the media and the courts, a circus of blame. There is always the fear that facts and innocence sell fewer newspapers than inflammatory headlines.

We had already contacted the detectives to initiate a homicide investigation. Lucky for all of us—the guy lived.

Long before you ever get involved in a self-defense situation, you have to lay a background. You need to know what your own ethical beliefs about violence entail and you need to understand the laws on using force.

Your ethical beliefs limit your behavior. Most people accept that killing is wrong, but understand that some other things are worse. When presented with something worse, like dying, killing seems less wrong. This line is blurry and different for each person. If you do not know where your line is, not just for killing but also for all the levels of force, you will freeze.

When someone is trying to kill you, you won't have time to work out your issues.

Laws set the standard for behavior and you will be held to it. You must know how the law limits what you can and cannot do—and then you must adapt your training to work within those limits.

Most martial artists train in systems that predate effective legal systems. Things that would have been acceptable in the Japan of the 1850s or during the Japanese occupation of Indonesia, Manchuria, or the Philippines will get you arrested and imprisoned today.

You need to know this stuff in advance so that you can be prepared.

1.1: legal (criminal)

Force law varies by state and sometimes, especially as it applies to weapons, by city. The principles are pretty universal but you need to personally read the statutes of your state. If you are a self-defense instructor, you need not only read them; but also to understand them, print them out, and have copies available to your students. Do a web search for your state and statutes or "revised statutes" and then search the statutes for "self-defense" and "force" and "justification." Printed copies of the criminal code and statutes for your state will also be available from your state government. READ THEM YOURSELF! If your on-line search through the statutes for self defense law comes up empty, it is possible that the state has not codified the law. Try a global search for "your state" + "self defense" + "jury instructions."

1.1.1: affirmative defense

The first thing you must understand is that in court self-defense is an *affirmative defense*. This has two huge implications. The first is that you are acknowledging the basic facts of what you did—if you hit someone with a brick and caused severe injury you are acknowledging that what you did falls under the definition of assault with a dangerous weapon and/or aggravated assault. Serious felonies. If your affirmative defense of self-defense does not work, you have effectively pled guilty. To claim self-defense is essentially saying, "Yes, I committed murder, but it was justified because . . ."

The second implication is that it puts the burden of proof on the defense. That's you. You have acknowledged the prosecutor's case. His work is done. By you. You now have to prove why, in your case, the brick assault was not bad. You have to prove why you had no choice. Prove. Beyond a reasonable doubt.

Defendants are not found guilty or innocent in a court of law. They are found guilty or not guilty. Guilty beyond a reasonable doubt, or not guilty because some doubt was achieved. To make an affirmative defense work you want to leave *no* doubt that your actions are justified.

1.1.2: elements of force justification

You must be able to explain, to a jury, what you did, why you did it, and why other choices would have been worse. This is difficult and it can take considerable practice to articulate in words a decision that happened in a fraction of a second. The law is the standard that you will be held to in the investigation. Your ethics are the standard that will control your actions in the moment.

Force justification is the science of explaining what you did.

First you must understand what you are allowed to do. The basic formula is:

"You may use the minimum level of force that you reasonably believe is necessary to safely resolve the situation."

Almost every part of that sentence is a legal concept. We'll go into more detail on the pieces later, but let's break it down.

". . . may use . . ." You are not required to use force. That's not your job. When this is presented to police officers the wording changes to "required." Officers have a duty to act and, generally, can't just walk away from a dangerous situation. You can, and you should walk away whenever possible.

". . . minimum level of force . . ." You can sort various types of force into rough categories. Deadly force, like a knife or a gun, are designed and intended to kill. Most blunt weapons like clubs, or attacking joints, are designed to injure. Sometimes you can cause pain with little risk of injury with a joint lock or a nerve pinch. Sometimes a push or a shout is all that is required. You will be required, if your actions go to court, to explain not only why you chose your course of action, but why a lesser level of force would not have worked.

". . . reasonably . . ." There is a lot of case law trying to define reasonable. In the end, the jury will determine if what you did was at the same level that someone else would have chosen. That imaginary someone will, theoretically, have the same training and experience as you. In reality, considering it is a jury of your peers, they will try to imagine if what you did was what they would have done.

". . . believe . . ." You will need to be able to articulate this, but legally you cannot be required to act on information you did not have. If a man says "I am going to kill you," and reaches for his waistband, you should be able to articulate why you believed he was going for a gun. You may find out later that he was reaching for a pack of gum and that he threatens to kill people all the time, but your belief in your own danger stemmed from what you saw and heard. To claim self-defense you must not only have felt threatened but also be able to explain to a jury why any other reasonable person would have *believed* he or she was in danger.

". . . is necessary . . ." You must prove that force was the only option. This is the one that gets the most effect from local law. In most states you will need to explain why you couldn't leave. Law aside; if you stay when you could have left after a verbal challenge or an argument, it wasn't self-defense. It was monkey dancing. A mutual fight. In other states with "stand your ground" laws it gets murkier. As it reads, you do not have to retreat even if retreat is an option. Legislators write the laws and they get recorded . . . and only later do we find out how the courts will interpret the law. I would hate to be the first test case at trial under a new "stand your ground" law.

". . . to safely . . ." This is a hard concept for people who were raised on John Wayne movies and martial sports. Self-defense is not a

States have different laws on requirements to claim self-defense. Some states are "duty to retreat"—they require you, in some cases, to exhaust all means of escape before you can attempt to defend yourself with force.

Many states have "castle laws" which lower the standards of proof in self-defense situations in the home. In essence, if you are attacked in your home or someone breaks into your house, Intents, Means and Opportunity are givens. A castle law, to a great extent, removes the Preclusion requirement.

A "stand-your-ground" law removes the preclusion requirement. Stand-your-ground law or not, it is prudent and probably critical to show that you attempted not to fight if you want to show self-defense.

contest. Fair play is not required by law. You don't use the minimum level of force that gives you a good chance of winning. You use the level of force, the minimum level of force, that you believe will get you out of the situation intact.

". . . resolve . . ." Resolving—ending—the situation is critical. But it may not be the resolution you envision. Getting out of there resolves the situation just as well as ending up with an unconscious bad guy. Think less about stopping the bad guy and more about getting to safety. Your safety is the goal, the optimal resolution. Do not lock-in, as many martial artists do, on the thought that stopping the Threat is the best or only way of achieving safety.

". . . the situation . . ." Sometimes the situation is obvious—an armed man threatening you and your loved ones while you are cornered in the back of a restaurant. Often things are less obvious—seeing someone break into your car while you are safely in your house. Seeing someone break into a stranger's car. The manager of a place you frequent asking someone to leave who refuses. The same manager asking for your help in bouncing the unruly patron. Voluntarily placing yourself in the situation usually excludes the affirmative defense of self-defense. Not always, though, if you are clearly seen by witnesses as someone trying to calm things down. In that case, that is still defending people. Defending property is more problematic. Read your own state statutes on that.

1.1.2.1: the threat

"Threat" is the law enforcement term for someone who requires officers to use force. The bad guy. If you use physical force to defend yourself, it will be on a Threat. You must be able to articulate why the person was a threat to you and how you knew it. Most people are good at reading other people, they get a feeling around dangerous people. However, "I had a feeling," won't cut it in court. You need to practice analyzing and explaining what causes your feelings.

In order to be a valid immediate threat, the individual must exhibit three things and another fourth element is necessary. These are Intent, Means, Opportunity and Preclusion.

Intent: The Threat must indicate to you, and you must be able to explain how you knew, that he wants to harm you. Sometimes it is obvious—"I'm going to kill you!" Sometimes slightly more subtle— three people spreading out to cut off your lines of retreat; an angry man suddenly going pale and gripping a beer bottle in a way better suited to swinging than swigging . . .

Means: Whatever the intent of the threat, he must have the means to carry out his intent. Sometimes that is size and fists or boots. If the Threat says, "I'm going to shoot you!" while wearing a bikini at the local swimming pool you will not be able to convince the jury you had to shoot her because you will not be able to convince the jury that you really believed she had a gun. An enraged six-year-old can have a lot of intent, but they are pretty lacking in means unless they get hold of a gun or a sharp knife. Or an ax. Maybe a chain saw.

Opportunity: The Threat must be able to reach you with the means. An unarmed Threat screaming outside your house cannot quickly get through the locked doors. He doesn't yet have opportunity. Your wife's loser ex may be a hardened felon with a thing for knives and guns but he won't have opportunity until he gets out of prison.

Once the Threat has shown Intent, Means, and Opportunity (IMO) he is a valid Threat and you are in danger. One other element should be satisfied for you to justify using force to defend yourself.

Preclusion: You must be able to convince a jury that you did not have any other viable option. You couldn't leave (e.g., Threat blocking the exit, helpless family left behind, or you had already tried to leave and he stopped you). You couldn't talk your way out (you tried and failed or maybe the Threat was screaming and howling too loud to listen) you couldn't call for help, or help would not arrive in time. You *must* be able to articulate why force was the one option that would safely work.

Those four elements: Intent, Means, Opportunity, and Preclusion, are the critical elements to justifying force.

1.1.3: scaling force

If a force incident lasts more than a few seconds, you must recognize that it is a very volatile situation. It changes quickly. This means that the four elements of Intent, Means, Opportunity, and Preclusion can also quickly change.

If you break the Threat's arm, you have hampered (but not eliminated) his Means. If, however, you break his arm and he falls to the floor crying and begging you to stop, you can bet that he has lost Intent. Once the Intent, Means, or Opportunity is gone, you are no longer defending yourself. Anything you do after that moment in time will be excessive force and possibly assault.

If your defense creates new opportunities for Preclusion, if for instance the Threat stumbles or you take him down, you may be able

More detail in the crime dynamics section, but if someone says, "Shut the fuck up or I'm going to beat your ass," and it escalates into a fight you will have real trouble proving self-defense . . . because you didn't simply shut the fuck up. Self-defense is about defending your body, not your pride. If this threat display devolves into a fight, you were engaged in the Monkey Dance. You were not defending yourself.

to leave. If you could safely leave and you don't, you have changed this from self-defense to a mutual fight and shattered your affirmative defense.

"... *to safely resolve the situation* ..." Changes as well. If your defense is effective, as you increase your control over the Threat or as the Threat takes damage, you should need less force. If you hit the Threat so hard that he is dizzy and can't see, a push may be enough to put him down or far enough away for you to escape to safety. If a push is enough, you don't use more.

If you arc losing, it is a pretty sure sign that you are *not* using enough force to safely resolve the situation. Losing is damage and damage diminishes your own Means. If it is an assault (mutual fighting is irrelevant to a discussion on self-defense), taking damage authorizes an increase in force. You have already proven that your first judgment of what would work safely was wrong.

There are many elements that will influence how much force is necessary. The size, strength, health and sometimes the age of the Threat matters, as well as your own size, strength and age. An unarmed six-year-old should not require as much force to restrain as an enraged linebacker.

Multiple threats will be a harder fight than a single threat. If someone brags about their combat skill, it is a clue not to wrestle with him or her and might justify going to a weapon of some kind immediately. If you are trapped—marched into an industrial freezer or pinned in a corner or thrown in a van or invaders are in your home—you have fewer options than if you had freedom to move. Fewer options often require greater force.

In certain cases the environment itself makes an encounter so dangerous that it must be ended quickly, and ending things quickly usually involves more force. Struggling next to a busy road or on a fire escape, for instance.

If you are surprised (see Section 4) that automatically justifies a very high level of force. You do not have time to gather enough information to accurately gauge an appropriate response. Time is damage in an ambush. You must shut down the threat to buy the time.

These are some of the elements that will affect what level of force you need. Making the decision is not enough. In order to prevail with a claim of self-defense you must be able to articulate (See Section 1.1.5) how these elements dictated your actions.

1.1.4: civil law

This will be a big part of the seventh section on post-conflict problems but the groundwork goes here.

There are two systems of justice in the United States. The criminal courts will determine if what you did was self-defense or a crime and whether you go home or to prison. Even if you prevail in criminal court you can be sued in civil court for the same event. It is not double jeopardy (wherein you cannot be tried twice for the same criminal offense). The purpose of civil court is not to determine whether you broke the law, but whether you are responsible for harm done to another person.

In a civil trial culpability is based not on "proof beyond a reasonable doubt," but by "the preponderance of the evidence." This means that if the jury believes that you are slightly more responsible than not, they may find against you.

The plaintiff (the person who is suing) must show that tangible harm was caused, and that you caused it. Tangible harm includes injuries that resulted in medical bills, lost work time, and loss of potential future earnings. Emotional distress has also been ruled, at times, to be a tangible harm.

In addition, the jury can award "punitive damages," an amount of money beyond the tangible losses of the plaintiff for the purpose of teaching you a lesson.

Because the burden of proof is lighter it is very possible to have a self-defense plea work in criminal court and still lose the civil case.

To prevail in a civil suit, you must convince the jury that the Threat left you no choice—that any harm he received was the result of *his* actions. To be absolved of responsibility you must show, absolutely, that the Threat was entirely responsible and it was pure self-defense.

Even if you prevail in criminal and civil court, it can be enormously expensive in time and money. Courts are a place for professionals, for lawyers. Self-defense law is a specialty.

I will give you some advice here, well aware that very few will actually follow it: research, get to know and consider putting a good attorney on retainer *now*. If you ever need an attorney, you will want one quickly and you will want a good one. It also tends to prevent police officers from making quick decisions when you have your attorney's card in your wallet.

1.1.5: articulation

Having all of the elements (Intent, Means, Opportunity, and Preclusion) is not enough to make your case. You must be able to explain to a jury and to investigators each element. It is always wisest to talk to investigators with your attorney present. Sometimes the events are clear. If a person shot the bank teller and the bank guard and then pointed his pistol at you, most juries would get that.

If three young men came up the parking garage stairs together, saw you and then began spreading-out, can you put into words why drawing a handgun was a good idea? You won't be explaining it to twelve men and women who studied self-defense. You will be explaining it to a jury who likely has no context or relative experience to bring to the decision. Your explanations must be clear and logical.

There is an exercise that I encourage and you will read about it in Section 3.1 when we discuss intuition and training intuition. The Articulation Exercise is simply to practice explaining your decisions,

In 2003, in Great Britain, a convicted burglar, Brendon Fearon, sued Tony Martin. Fearon had broken into Martin's home and he and his accomplice were shot. The accomplice died, Fearon was wounded. Among the claims in the court proceedings was a claim for "loss of earnings." Fearon dropped the case in exchange for Martin dropping his counter-suit.

hunches, and conclusions. People rarely deal with or even think in facts. We spend a lot of time with conclusions.

"This was a great day," is not a fact; it is a conclusion. It's probably a conclusion based on a lot of little facts. Maybe you always feel better when it is sunny and windy, or after a great workout or when you get some unexpected praise. Usually it is a combination of many small things.

On a personal level, this practice teaches you how you work on the inside. Sometimes it will surprise you.

"He's a jerk," is not a fact, but a conclusion. It may be based on many little things: he acts like he is an old friend and we just met, he double-dips his chips in the shared ranch dressing; he tries to be bossy about things he doesn't know. This again, tells you a lot about yourself. What you dislike, what pushes your buttons. Once you realize the little behaviors that make someone a jerk you can start monitoring them in your own behavior. Very powerfully, you can look beyond them and start to see that mannerisms may be social incompetence hiding a decent person.

You will also learn to be more careful with some words. Good and bad are value judgments (conclusions) and I tend to avoid them. If I label someone as "bad," I know my own meaning: he will hurt someone to get what he wants. If I use "evil" it means he will hurt someone even when he doesn't want anything.

In making a case for self-defense, this practice is invaluable. Your knowledge of violence dynamics (Section 2) and your skills at observation and articulation will make your case.

What observations justify your alert to the three young men who come up the stairs together, see a lone person and spread out? Friends walking together walk together, they do not split off. Spreading-out cut off my lines of retreat. The fact that they didn't speak to each other after spotting me indicated that they had done this before.

1.2: ethics

Hurting someone else, the intentional infliction of pain and damage, is generally wrong. Invading another's space violates social taboos you have absorbed since childhood. Most of the rules you learned about how to be a good human involved not hurting people. Most of these rules are ingrained so deeply that you are not consciously aware of them.

If you ever need to defend yourself with force, you will likely run into these issues. What are your personal ethics of violence?

This is deep stuff, because what the conscious mind believes often has little bearing on what the person can do. It is perfectly logical to say, "I am willing to use deadly force to defend myself or my loved ones from imminent death or serious bodily injury." It's a nice statement. Very logical. Legally defensible. Clearly right on many levels.

Saying it does not mean you will do it.

In "Betrayed by the Angel" (*Harvard Review* Nov./Dec. 2004) Debra Anne Davis writes with heart-breaking honesty about her rape. I use her example, not because the situation is unique, but because her courage in writing about it is so rare.

In her description she tells of what I would call "decision points," e.g., "My first impulse is to shut the door. But I stop myself: You can't do something like that. It's rude." or "I've made the mental choice to be rude, but I haven't been able to muster the physical bluntness the act requires." At each of those decision points she did not make the decision based on the circumstances she faced. She made those decisions based on her self-image and early civilized programming.

She did not slam the door in her rapist's face because to do so would be rude.

Do not for one second think that this is uniquely her problem. Your programming is just as deep. The thoughts that "That would be rude" or "This kind of thing doesn't happen to people like me" are very common in people who suffer violent attacks and freeze.

This programming is subconscious and takes a great deal of work and insight to bring out into the light of day and consciously examine. It is imperative to work it out in advance.

1.2.1: the conscious stuff: capacity

Mauricio Machuca, a friend and martial arts instructor in Montreal, talks about *capability* and *capacity*. Capability is a physical skill. If you are a martial artist you know how to hurt another human being. That is one of your capabilities. But not everyone is emotionally equipped to hurt a human being. It doesn't always come out in the knowledge: "I could never do that. It's wrong." More often it comes out when you actually apply fingers to flesh and begin to twist, even in training, and feel a sinking in your gut. When the idea of putting your fingers through someone's eyes creeps you out. That is capacity, and not everyone has the internal, personal capacity to inflict harm on another person.

I don't know where your capacity lies. In all likelihood, neither do you. I know quite a bit about mine but I doubt if I truly know the limits. I know what I have done to violent criminals when I was at risk. I'm okay with that. But change an element . . .

Let's play a game:

Someone comes at you with a butcher knife. You have nowhere to retreat. You have a gun. The Threat has Intent, Means, and Opportunity to kill you and you have precluded all other options. This is a shoot/no-shoot scenario. Do you shoot? Do you kill? Are you okay with that? Think about it.

Now change an element. The Threat is twelve years old. Do you still shoot? Kill? Are you okay with that?

If the Threat were six years old? Four?

A woman?

A pregnant woman?

A mentally disabled person who can't realize what they are doing?

Your own spouse?

Your own child?

> Everything in this book affects everything else. Working out your internal ethics well in advance vastly eases the effects of certain types of freezes that will be discussed in Section 5.

13

What if the Threat's toddler children are watching?

What if cameras are rolling?

The threat is the same—even a four-year-old with a big knife can kill and there are no degrees of dead. Do you feel the same about all of those scenarios? I don't. Even knowing full well how dangerous a knife is and how many people die from overconfidence I would have a hard time shooting a child. I might feel differently about the other scenarios but would act the same—I would just feel worse about it later.

Think about this. Explore it. Listen to your gut feelings before you try to logic it out. When you do try to logic it out, pay special attention to when you are rationalizing—when your logic is serving not to make the best decision but to justify the decision that your gut wants.

That is bad logic, but it is not a bad thing. Your gut knows you better than your brain ever will. Your training should align itself with your gut.

If the age of the Threat matters, you might have a bigger concern with appearing to be too weak to deal with a "small problem." You, to some degree, might value your ego over your life. (S'okay. We all do that to some degree.)

Gender doesn't matter much with a knife. Dead is dead and the point of a knife is that it doesn't take strength to leave you bleeding on the floor. If you hesitate here, you may be crippled by your own macho self-image.

If your gut clenched on the pregnant woman, you are aware that your actions will also impact people you can't see. This is just basic sensitivity, even wisdom . . . but it can kill you. Wise isn't always safe.

If you would have trouble shooting the mentally disabled, you have the two concepts of self-defense and justice intertwined. You want whatever force you use to be used on someone who is bad or, preferably, evil. That does make the conscience easier. Unfortunately, you can be hurt or killed by people who may not be able to understand the ramifications of what they do.

Using deadly force against family brings up all kinds of cognitive dissonance. If you are willing to die to protect someone, where is the line between that and letting someone kill you so that you don't kill them? Objectively, mathematically, they are the same, but someone trying to kill you is not the family member you imagine. A low-level version of this may explain why date rape so rarely inspires violent physical resistance.

If you hesitate with toddlers watching you, know that what you do in this arena will have ripples forever. It is easy to talk about killing, but some people wince when you say "manufacturing corpses" or "converting a person to meat." They physically shrink back when you use the words, "making widows and orphans."* Widows and orphans. People with no culpability who will be forever changed by your actions.

If cameras bother you it *may* be because you doubt your own judgment or have insecurities that you will do the right thing. More likely you understand that any use of force appears shocking to most citizens. No matter how justified a killing, if it makes good news it will be broadcast and draw comments. If it excites more people to portray you as the villain then that is the way you will be portrayed.

This is the type of stuff that you can work out by logic, sometimes. And sometimes you can change it by logic and insight. Sometimes. Section 1.2.1.1 is a tool that may help you work some things out.

1.2.1.1: beliefs, values, morals and ethics

I learned this paradigm at the Academy two decades ago and I have no idea who invented it. (See Fig. 1-001.) If a reader does, let me know. The original authors deserve a lot of credit.

People have a hierarchy of understanding and behavior—things that drive what they do, say, and *are*.

At the lowest level of the hierarchy are *beliefs*. These are simply the things you hold to be true. These are not necessarily objective truths (diamond is harder than chalk) but often subjective truths: One can believe with absolute sincerity that the world is flat or round; that God does or does not exist; that people are basically good or basically

---

* I speak harshly on this, particularly in person, because I don't want people to EVER gloss over the profound cost of taking a life. If you can just say 'dead' or 'kill' without grasping the repercussions then it allows you to indulge in bullshit macho fantasies. The fantasies do not help—they set one up for failure.

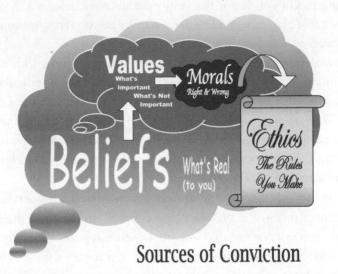

Fig. 1-001: Hierarchy of Understanding Behavior

When my children were very young, I found that I was getting risk adverse, hesitating (minimally, but still there) on taking chances even when they were necessary and right. It may sound stupid, but a solid life insurance policy that made sure my family would be financially okay—pay off my home, cover kids' college, and complete living expenses for four years—helped remove a developing glitch.

selfish. Beliefs are our internal assumptions about the world and they lay the foundation for everything we do and say.

The next level up is *values*. Of all the things that we believe, some are more important than others. If you believe that God only allows prayer for healing and you believe that your child will die without an operation, which choice do you make? If you believe that politeness is critical to society but also believe that a certain individual only responds to anger, what do you do? You can see values in actions far more easily than in words. Beliefs and values, generally, are very deeply planted and not conscious at all.

Morals derive from values and are your vague gut-level feelings about what is right and wrong. All of the things that you "just know are wrong" without being able to explain why constitute your morals.*

Ethics are your personal code, the general rules that you make up for yourself to try to put your morals into words.

This is an aside, but this model has worked brilliantly for me in resolving disputes and understanding disagreements. In disagreements, the deeper the level the more difficult the argument. A disagreement at the ethics level, for instance, can be friendly.

As an example, two people can disagree on whether the list of the levels of force discussed above is complete. One may be happy with it while another wants to distinguish between pure pain such as pressure points, and techniques such as locks, which threaten injury. The ethics level is the most conscious, which lends to reasoned discourse, but it is also the least personal. An argument at the ethics level is not perceived as an attack on identity.

An argument at the belief level, however, is very much an attack on identity. Arguing religion or politics, according to research, stimulates the emotional, not the logical parts of the brain. Telling someone one of their beliefs is wrong is telling them that they are stupid. It will be perceived as a personal attack.

The abortion debate in the US, for example, stems from the belief level but is argued usually at the value level. If you believe that the fetus is a human, there are few if any possible values higher than the innocent life of a child. If you do not believe this, the debate is entirely one of a piece of tissue versus the coercion of a woman.

You cannot successfully argue (or even really understand) from a higher level than the core disbelief. If someone disagrees with you at the belief level, you cannot convince him or her at any higher level.

If you can explain yourself from a deeper level you are far more likely to get the other person to comprehend your point of view.

---

* The language here is specific to this model. In fact, morals and ethics are merely the Latin and Greek translations of each other. The model requires a distinction between this level and the next.

Ethics are the easiest to alter. We have all played a game, consciously or not, where someone makes a blanket statement and we come up with objections, obscure "what-ifs" where the rule doesn't hold.

"Thou shalt not kill" is a simple ethic. It is based on the moral that killing is wrong, on the value that life is important, and on the belief that both life and death exist.

Morally, it can be argued that there are different types of killing with different moral weights. Self-defense is different than beating someone to death for his wallet. Ergo, self-defense, killing for food (since even plants are alive), etc., are moral arguments that dispute a simple ethic.

At the value level, most people accept that there are some things more important than an individual human life. Was demolishing the institution of slavery sufficient justification for the deaths lost in the Civil War? Was stopping Hitler or Napoleon worth the lives that those wars cost? Someone thought that twenty million executions in Russia was a small price to pay for the Revolution. Would you sacrifice your own life to save ten children from a spree murderer? Would you kill the spree murderer?

At the belief level it is much more difficult to make change. You can possibly bring out contradictory beliefs, e.g., "If you believe that life is eternal, it's impossible to kill in any case." Or you can attack the epistemology.

Epistemology is how a person or society decides what is true. Tradition, the stories of the Shamans, or reading it in Popular Science can all be epistemologies. I mentioned the flat/round earth belief above, think about this:

Is the Earth round? Yes, of course. However, most people have no direct knowledge of the facts that lead to this conclusion or even a vague idea of how to go about proving it to their satisfaction. They believe the Earth is round because they were told by people they trusted. It is, for most people, a subjective truth and no more based on fact than the belief that the world is held up by four elephants standing on the back of an enormous turtle. If you were to backtrack this belief to its source, you would know much about how you were raised to believe things, the epistemology of your society.

Thus ends the aside. That was about applying this tool, Belief Values Morals and Ethics (BVME) to others. You can also apply it to yourself to change your capacity.

The gut feelings in the exercise above found your resistance at the moral level. You will not be able to change these beliefs with a logical (ethical-level) argument. The deeper you can challenge your resistance, the more successful you will be.

One example that has worked very, very well for me is the value that I place on my own children. I can't think of much that I value higher. I have risked, and would probably give my life to prevent a death, to prevent children I did not know from losing a father. Would I hesitate to defend myself to protect these unseen children?

From the ethical level, doing the math and saying the words, it's a wash. What I say I value and what I say I am willing to pay work out the same either way. Someone dies, some orphans are created, and other orphans are prevented.

The moral level is indignant. Hell no. That bastard is the one who decided to create this situation. I'd much rather have a world without the likes of him in it than without the likes of me. It's good at the moral level, powerful but . . .

His kids become orphans or my kids? No-brainer. My kids will not be orphans, ever, if I have anything to say about it.

If you can track your hesitations down to the value level, you can institute some profound change. However, it is not really change, but simply clarity. Your values don't change, you have just worked out things in advance that would take time when you are under attack. You won't have time then. You do have time now. In self-defense, clarity adds speed.

1.2.2: the unconscious stuff: finding your glitches

In my own experience, almost everyone hesitates before doing a dangerous or uncomfortable thing. Whether jumping out of an airplane or diving into cold water or singing karaoke in public, very few people can just go for it without hesitation the first time.

This is troubling, because I can guarantee that if you are about to get into a fight it will be unpleasant and uncomfortable and frightening. Even more so if you have never done it before. That's a recipe for hesitation. If you are attacked, every second of hesitation is a second of damage. The longer the hesitation lasts the more damage you take the less able you become to do anything effective when and if you do act. That is some pretty cold math. Section 5 on Breaking the Freeze will go into more detail on how to act. Here we need to talk about finding some of your glitches.

First and foremost you must practice noticing your own hesitations, no matter how minor. You WILL have a tendency to rationalize them, to say, "That wasn't a hesitation, that was just a stutter." It's the same. This is deep stuff, some of it going to the very core of your identity. You will subconsciously throw up resistance to anything that threatens your identity—even new, good information. Even growth.

Notice when you hesitate. Ideally, you will have friends and coaches watching for the same things. This is something that I, as a self-defense instructor, specialize in catching—not just the big, overt hesitations but the narrowing eyes that come with an unwelcome thought or the quicker breathing when trying to deny something unpleasant. Look for those signs in yourself . . . and do not rationalize them.

One example that will be familiar to most martial artists: two students practicing at light or no contact and one accidentally hits the other in the face. Even with a light touch, both of their eyes go wide, both take a step back, hands go up and the apologies start to spew.

Does this make any sense at all? Two people studying martial arts (arts dedicated to Mars, the god of war) specifically in a class where one of the seeming goals is to learn how to hit people . . . and there is an immediate, visceral and almost universal reaction to face contact.

The glitch here comes from one of our greatest social taboos: adults do not touch other adults on the head. It is okay to pat a child on the head, or to touch a lover's face. That's a short list. To touch another adult on the head is extremely insulting, a sign of great intimacy or great domination. It is, in normal situations, "simply not done."

That's a problem, especially if what you have learned for self-defense involves hitting people in the face.

You find these glitches and you get past them most effectively by repeated exposure. At a minimum level, get used to face contact, and taking hits. Some go much farther and there is something feral and dangerous about the person who has experienced enough contact that getting tagged in the face means the training is going to be fun today.

Face contact is an obvious, easy-to-see glitch that almost everyone has. I don't know where the rest of your glitches are. I don't know which of my own glitches I have yet to discover. That's just the way it is. You can't truly know your limits, physically or emotionally, until you've reached them. Go to your limits enough, however, and they move.

There is one other exercise I would like to suggest. If you know or can get to know someone who raises livestock, slaughter an animal.

It may sound horrible, and that is the point. Hunting is not the same: you are the predator and using a bow or a rifle, the kill is at a distance. Slaughtering using a knife (I have done it using a sword) is *killing*, close and personal and messy. You will feel and see the life leave the animal's body and eyes. It is a little piece of something you might experience if you ever have to defend yourself. Killing an animal will not have the same emotional weight as killing a person, but you might be shocked by the impact it has on you. That's good. Consider it a vaccination, a slight bit of dealing with the glitch so that you will be strong enough to handle it if or when the real thing comes along.

1.2.3: through the looking glass*

This is yet another concept that will come up again in "Breaking the Freeze."

Glitches are not new to you. You have dealt all your life with learning to do things that weren't easy for you; doing things that made you nervous or queasy; overcoming imaginary limitations. From the third-grader who decides that she can't learn cursive, to the person who learned to drive even though they swore weren't mechanically inclined. In your life you have faced a lot of glitches and either gotten over them or decided to live with them.

The glitches in a self-defense situation will be qualitatively different because of the stakes, the time, and inexperience.

The grade school student who decides she can't do fractions is at most risking a bad grade or being teased by her friends or chastised by her parents. The college student who chokes on a test may be risking a career. The person who chokes in a sudden attack will cross the line from survivor to victim. The stakes are high: life, health, and even identity.

If you started out like many baby-boomers, saying, "I'm not computer savvy," you have had years to get over it. Plenty of time to learn the basics and even develop a little skill, no matter how confused you were the first time you heard the word DOS (if you don't know what that is, ask your parents). In a sudden attack, you will have little or no time to work out your glitches, your ethical issues, your capacities. Whatever time it takes will cost you in damage. That is why it is imperative to work out all you can well in advance of any attack.

Lastly, very few people have extensive experience with violence. Two shoot-outs may total fewer than thirty seconds of experience. Hundreds of brawls barely means a few hours of experience, most of that jacked-up on adrenaline. And what you know from your peaceful world does not apply in the world of violence.

Stakes, time, and experience.

---

* This is a reference to the Lewis Carroll sequel to *Alice in Wonderland* (1892). It is shorthand for being in a place where the rules are all very different.

You have been raised with specific attitudes, beliefs, and tactics to handle confrontation. They have centered on dealing with playground and possibly corporate bullies, dinner table arguments with family, and dominance games at work. That is conflict in the civilized world and you have tactics for that. The world of violence where one person puts hands or weapons on another to cause harm is not typically a part of that world.

The beliefs and attitudes that *prevent* normal people from physically attacking are not present in the world of violence, so why would you think the tactics that work in the boardroom would be successful here?

Our normal defensive strategies and skills for dealing with conflict may be one of the very factors that work against us in a fight. These skills have been honed over a lifetime and they are efficient and well-practiced and trusted, and they are keyed to an environment and a specific society.

For most women, for most people, these defenses are social. They are ways of avoiding confrontation, not ways to resolve violence. Ignoring. Appeasement. Flattery. Self-deprecation. "I'm on your side"—teaming.

When the environment changes from a social situation where conflict is pending to a violent or predatory situation where the battle is on, every single one of these sets the victim up for failure, more clearly labels the victim as a *victim*. Possibly worse, when it is all over and the bruises have healed, these failed strategies will be remembered as cowardice or compliance, and compound the survivor guilt until, tragically, the victim may even convince herself that she deserved or wanted the attack.

The very unfamiliarity of violence can be one of the biggest glitches of all.

I tell you now, the dark side of the looking glass is one of the environments you have evolved to deal with. It doesn't have to be a glitch. You do have to give yourself permission to quit being a nice person and start being an effective animal.

CHAPTER 2: VIOLENCE DYNAMICS

Bill and I were talking to the warden in an Iraqi prison, drinking chai. A gun fired. Other than ours and the warden's bodyguards, there shouldn't have been loaded weapons in that section of the building. I put down my tea, stood and drew my sidearm. I started clearing the building. Slow is smooth, smooth is fast.

Button hooking each door, scanning the room, "Clear!" Bill was right behind me. Everything seemed slow, but no one else had begun to react yet. I realized that nothing was happening. Hordes of well-armed militia were not pouring into the corridor. There was no second shot.

Animals are social creatures. Even as they broke out of the freeze one-by-one, they weren't running away from the shot. Neither were they gathering around to watch. The behavior of the others told me long before I got to the end of the corridor that it was neither an assault, a gunfight, nor even a suicide. I knew it was an accidental discharge before I turned into the last room.

I cleared the weapon, comforted the poor guy in a language I barely understood and left it for the warden to handle. Then I went back to finish my tea.

Understanding violence can be extremely complex. As a subject, violence could be said to extend from toddlers wrestling to boxing to rape to nuclear war. Self-defense, however, fits in a narrower range and this chapter will study the dynamics of the violence where self-defense is appropriate—criminal violence.

Generally, violence can be broken down into two very broad categories: social and asocial.

Social violence is what, in the natural world, would be the types of violence common within a single species. This intra-species violence does not follow the dynamic or use the same tactics as violence against other species. The dominance game of snakes wrestling or bears pushing and mouthing is not the same as the way the same species hunt prey.

Social violence includes ritualized jockeying for territory or status. It also includes acts to prove or increase group solidarity (a powerful side-effect of hunting as a team) and violence to enforce the rules and mores of the group.

Asocial violence does not target the victim as a person, but as a resource. Asocial violence is the domain of the predator and the humanity of his victim does not enter into the equation.

What follows are descriptions. How to deal with these dynamics is the subject of Chapter Three.

2.1: social violence

Social violence can roughly be delineated as the Monkey Dance (MD), the Group Monkey Dance (GMD), the Educational Beat-Down (EBD) and the Status-Seeking Show (SSS).

2.1.1: the monkey dance

Most, if not all animals have a ritualized combat between males of the same species to safely establish dominance. Snakes coil around each other and wrestle. It can look like mating to the uninitiated. Deer and elk lock antlers and push and fence. Rams slam their horns, reinforced with massive blocks of bone, into each other. Humans fist-fight or wrestle.

In all cases, it is a ritual with specific steps, genetically designed NOT to be life-threatening.

This human dominance game, the Monkey Dance, follows specific steps. (See Fig. 2-001.) You have all seen it:

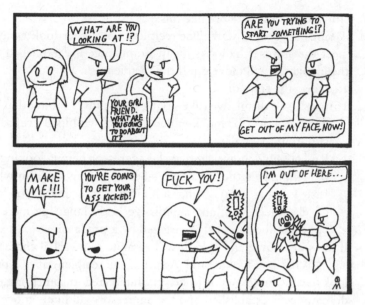

Fig. 2-001: The Basic Monkey Dance

1) A hard, aggressive stare
2) A verbal challenge, e.g., "What you lookin' at?"
3) An approach, often with the signs of increased adrenaline: gross motor activity of arm swinging or chest bobbing, a change in color, usually with the skin flushing.
4) As the two square-off, there may be more verbal exchanges and then one will make contact. It will usually be a two-handed push on the chest or an index finger to the chest. If it is an index finger to the nose (remember face contact, above) it will go immediately to step #5. If there is no face contact, this step can be repeated many times until one of the dancers throws . . .
5) A big, looping over-hand punch.

This description is simplified and shows only one side. It must be emphasized that there have been thousands of generations conditioned to play this game in this way. It is easy to get sucked in and a very difficult thing to walk away. Backing down from a Monkey Dance, unless you take or are given a face-saving out, is extremely difficult and embarrassing, especially for young men.

A full MD will look more like this:

1) A hard, aggressive stare. The recipient will either look away or meet the stare. If he looks away, dominance is established and the instigator will move on. If the recipient:

1a) meets the stare or

1b) tries to be dismissive (like saying to friends, "I think that guy has the 'hots' for me"), either of which will likely cause the situation to escalate.

1c) It is possible, however, that the aggressor here is looking for or willing to settle for a Status-Seeking Show (SSS) in which case looking away, being submissive, may mark you as a good target. Also, any submissive body language increases your likelihood of being targeted by a predator.

2) If the stare is met and held, it will escalate to a verbal challenge, e.g., "What you lookin' at?" Again, if the recipient at this point looks away and pretends to be very interested in something else, dominance is established and the aggressor will likely move on. The recipient, especially if girls are watching, will have an incredible urge to respond in kind. It is, in fact, fear of being humiliated by not responding that is driving the dynamic. The MD is not a game you play. It is genetically programmed and unless you possess wisdom and exert will, the game plays *you*.

2a) In order to defuse, the looking away must be submissive. It must be humble. If the recipient looks away but starts snickering with friends or making low-voiced comments, the verbal challenge is repeated and escalated, "Hey! Asshole! I'm talking to you!"

2b) If the recipient is not feeling submissive and is not mature enough to avoid the MD, he answers the verbal response. "Who's asking?"

3) An approach, often marked by adrenalin-linked signs: gross motor activity of arm swinging or chest bobbing; a change in color, usually with the skin flushing.

3a) At this point, other monkeys get involved. Friends of both sides try to intervene, get between the two and prevent any further escalation. This is one of the best ways to have a face-saving resolution. No one is injured, no one backed down. Status is not established but the willingness to fight for status has been, no matter how easy it was for bystanders to separate the dancers. This sets boundaries and allows both to co-exist with mutual respect, one of the main goals of the Monkey Dance.

3b)If one of the dancers is alone, he now has the face-saving exit in that he is not backing down from the opponent, but from the group. If the lone person does not back down, it is probably a special case and will likely end very badly.*

3c) If no intervention is forthcoming, and again, especially if girls are watching, things will escalate to step 4.

4) As the two square-off there may be more verbal attacks and then one will make contact. It will usually be a two-handed push on the chest or an index finger to the chest. If it is an index finger to the nose (remember face contact, above) it will go immediately to Step #5. This pushing, with low-level contact can go on for some time. Marc MacYoung** pointed out that you will often see an approach/retreat body language where one of the dancers steps forward and makes contact, then steps back, hoping the other will back down.

5) A big, looping over-hand punch. At this point the fight, such as it is, will be on.

Get this—no matter who issued the verbal challenge, who pushed first or who threw the first punch there is no self-defense here. With all of the opportunities for preclusion, for *not* joining in the Monkey Dance, for simply leaving, this will be classified as a mutual combat fight. Both parties may go to jail. One certainly will if a serious injury results—even if it was from stumbling and falling.

---

* "Special cases" are individuals to whom many of the rules don't apply. These include people who choose to act crazy whenever threatened, experienced loners from violent backgrounds who can only imagine high levels of violence, and those so poorly socialized that they are conflicted in how to play the MD or even whether they are playing it. The point of this section is for you to understand the normal so that you can recognize the special cases.
** MacYoung.

Serious injuries are rare in the MD—the skull is designed to take damage from the front and hand bones are fragile. When an injury occurs it is usually either a fracture of the metacarpals or from someone falling and hitting his head. If that should happen and you should be charged with manslaughter, self-defense will not fly in court.

The Monkey Dance is very much a male ritual. It is a contest for status between males. Women, generally, do not feel the male fear that others will see them as wimps for not playing. And guys, for the record most women see backing down as mature and not cowardly (with thanks to the movie, "Support Your Local Sheriff".)

Very rarely a man will perceive himself to be in a Monkey Dance with a woman. This is another special case. It indicates a man who has not been properly socialized at all, has likely picked a woman out of desperation to be of superior status to *somebody* and can become dangerously enraged if the woman is not submissive—and sexually predatory if she is.

Special cases aside, the MD is almost always initiated with a person that the aggressor sees as close to his social level. In other words, a normal person will not follow the steps of the MD with a child. There is no status to be gained and the very idea that you thought that there might places you in a very low status.

Nor will a normal person MD with a very high-ranking individual, like a mob boss. Captains are constantly jockeying for influence, but they don't do it with generals and only the very insecure do it with lieutenants. Middle management is a hotbed of one-upmanship and subtle challenges, but the middle managers don't MD with the boss and the few that do MD with the line staff are the kind of managers that both make life hell and are the source of thousands of jokes.

2.1.2: the group monkey dance

The Group Monkey Dance (GMD) is a show of group solidarity. There are two levels, at least. In the lowest level an outsider is discouraged from interfering with group business—it is a way of establishing territory.

Families are tight-knit groups. Domestic violence incidents are acts within the group. Sometimes, when the police intervene, both parties turn on them. Even though one was a victim just moments before and in fear for her life, husband and wife, attacker and victim, often band together to drive away the outsiders.

This is behavior that is familiar in chimps and baboons—your tribe will band together to drive away or scare off members of another tribe or a predator. If you don't play, your loyalty to the group might be questioned.

In the higher level of GMD the victim is sometimes an outsider but often an insider who is perceived in some way to have betrayed the group. The group bands together in an orgy of violence, possibly beating, burning and cutting on the victim. It is literally a contest to show your loyalty by how much damage you can do to the outsider. Some of the most brutal murders, lynchings, and war atrocities are examples of the Group Monkey Dance.

Most GMDs occur when an outsider is within the threat-group's territory. There is an exception. You may remember the wildings in Central Park or the roving band of young men randomly beating people in Seattle. This pack behavior follows a similar dynamic and serves the same purpose as any other GMD—it strengthens bonds within the group. Causing fear in others (and fear is power) is just a by-product.

In earlier societies, this bonding-through-violence was ensured by hunting large game animals.

2.1.3: the educational beat-down

Most of the people reading this will be comfortable products of comfortable homes with significant education and socialization. This is the norm in North America, where I happen to be writing. The norm is so powerful and pervasive that it can be very easy to believe that the values of middle-class Americans are universal. They are not. There are societies and sub-societies where violence is merely an easy way to solve problems; where a beating is considered as easy and more effective than talking.

There are places in the United States where if you do something rude and improper you will get disapproving looks and people will whisper about you. They might snub you in the coffee room or not invite you to go bowling. And there are places in the US where doing something that society considers rude will get you beaten without a second thought.

If that is news to you, take a second and let it seep in.

Once upon a time, an inmate was beaten in one of the dorms at my jail. I was called to investigate. The dorm housed 65 inmates in an open bay (no cells) and the man had been hit in the center of the day room while watching TV. He looked to have only been hit twice—a bloody nose and a black eye.

I was pretty good at investigations. The inmates knew and trusted me and in most "nobody saw nothing" situations I would have the attacker identified and removed in under an hour. This time nobody was talking. They didn't seem angry or afraid, more . . . embarrassed.

I talked to the victim. He wouldn't tell me who hit him, of course. What he did say was, "Sarge, I had it coming. I forgot where I was. I was watching TV and I said, 'Hey, look, you could kill three niggers with one bullet.' Next thing I knew I was lying on my back. I deserved it." He looked me right in the eye, "It was sort of an educational beat-down," he said.

He was able to return to the dorm with no problem. The message had been sent and he showed that he had received it. His behavior was, to his peers' satisfaction, corrected.

In certain groups, *this is normal*. A casual beating is how rules are enforced and community standards, such as they are, are upheld.

Generally, if you were stupid and should have known better the Educational Beat Down will be quick, sometimes just a single strike, almost off-hand. It is the exact same thing as when a character in a comedy thwacks another on the head, only with a bit more intent. It is a spanking between adults.

If the recipient of the EBD acknowledges that they were wrong, (unless the transgression was particularly egregious—for instance in certain societies it would be the duty of the brothers to kill a sister's rapist), it is over quickly.

If the victim does not acknowledge that they broke a rule, if they argue or get indignant, then the assault will escalate. The person who delivers the Educational Beat Down is usually a respected member of the group. This is not a Monkey Dance, with two young puppies wrestling for dominance. This is a lesson, with the big dog batting the puppy to the floor and maybe pinning it there. (Still, it is not the same as predation, not in people or dogs.)

Not acknowledging the transgression sends the message that the victim does not acknowledge the Big Dog's status. It is taken as a clear indicator that he either does not know or does not care about the rules and must be taught a lesson. The damage will escalate until the transgressor/victim acknowledges that the message has been received. That acknowledgement must be free of excuses.

Another circumstance where the EBD will escalate is when the lesson is less for the transgressor than for everyone else. On May 7, 1929 Al Capone had Albert Anselmi, Joseph Giunta, and John Scalise tied to their chairs. He then beat them with a baseball bat and had them shot in the head. The lesson taught and the message delivered wasn't for Al, Joe, and John. It was for everyone else. Dead people don't learn anything.

This escalation can be extremely violent and occurs most often, and slightly less predictably, when the Big Dog is insecure in his status as leader or elder.

2.1.4: the status seeking show

If a young Threat brutally beats a foreign tourist in a random explosion of violence . . . it wasn't random. It was just a surprise for the onlookers and the victim.

In a marginal society, like the criminal subculture, a reputation for violence is a very valuable thing. If people think you are crazy, apt to "go-off" they treat you with more deference, fear to push your buttons. It is the perfect example of Machiavelli's observations on fear and love—both are nice, but if you have to pick one it is better to be feared than to be loved:

"Upon this a question arises: whether it be better to be loved than feared or feared than loved? It may be answered that one should wish to be both, but, because it is difficult to unite them in one person, it is much safer to be feared than loved, when, of the two, either must be dispensed with. Because this is to be asserted in general of men, that they are ungrateful, fickle, false, cowardly, covetous, . . . and men have less scruple in offending one who is beloved than one who is feared, for love is preserved by the link of obligation which, owing to the baseness of men, is broken at every opportunity for their advantage; but fear preserves you by a dread of punishment which never fails."—Nicolo Machiavelli, *The Prince* [*]

So how does one safely get this reputation? Beating on your allies, your own group, is rarely conducive to having them watch your back. It is counter-productive and dangerous, except at the very top of the social strata. The Big Dog, however, already has the reputation and actually puts his power in doubt by needing to show it.

Beating on enemies would work, but members of other groups have friends and, sometimes, long memories. That could easily escalate well beyond what you are prepared to deal with or want.

So how about victimizing someone traveling alone, or at least with no large male companions? An outsider but not an enemy. A relatively easy mark . . .

Understand this—the Status-Seeking Show can violate almost all of the rules of normal social violence and that is the point. The SSSer is trying to show his craziness, his willingness to break social rules. So they won't necessarily attack someone of their own social level (the norm in the Monkey Dance). Beating a child or woman shows craziness; beating a superior—like shooting a cop or ambushing the boss, is taken as both crazy and brave, no matter how safely the ambush was set up.

They also have no need to follow the steps of the Monkey Dance by issuing a challenge. The SSS is not limited in damage like the normal MD, either. A savage beating, knifing, or killing all satisfy the Threat's purpose.

[*] Machiavelli.

Understand this—each type of violence serves a purpose. It might make no sense according to the way that you look at the world, but your worldview is small and limited and, most importantly, does not matter when someone is trying to kill you. The Threat's worldview is the one that is calling the tune.

2.1.5: territory defense

Defending common territory is a hallmark of any group, whether an army, a tribe, or a troop of monkeys. Humans have expanded this idea and symbolized it in that many are willing to fight and die for intangibles—a flag, patriotism, a place in heaven. Just because the territory being defended or invaded is imaginary does not make the passion of the defenders any less.

Territory defense can also be very logical. From cowboys fighting for water rights to modern drug organizations fighting for market share, in areas where the law is weak, as in the Old West; or not an option because you really can't report that someone stole your illegal drugs, individuals and groups will defend their own things in their own way.

How violent the defense (or offense) may depend on the ability to "other" the opponent. As we will discuss with predators, most normal people cannot kill another human being in cold blood. Many cannot shoot even in war; some can't kill to defend their own lives. Much of the conditioning of soldiers and the bonding in other social sets serves the purpose of making it easier to see the enemy as "other": not us, not like us, maybe not even human.

If you can convince yourself that you are killing animals, you are more free to use the tactics, tools, and mindset of killing animals and less likely to fall prey to the conscience and psychological damage of killing your fellow human. Even if you can't go that far, can't convince yourself that they are only animals, if you can only convince yourself that they are very different, they no longer have the right to the courtesy—the warnings, the challenge or the mercy—that you would extend to a member of your own group.

It is possible that the gangs I worked with in the jails were broken down along racial lines because it is easier to "other" people who look different than people who look like you. That "othering" makes you a bit quicker to resort to violence and more brutal with the violence that you do apply. There are other factors at play of course—crime tends to be run along friendship and kin lines and through neighborhoods—but "othering" and its ability to make quick harsh violence easier is an advantage.

Territory defense is the bridge between social and asocial violence. It is profoundly social—defending the group, the group's home, the group's resources—but is often carried out in a manner that is profoundly asocial. This is a situation deliberately created and maintained by the leaders and elders of the involved group. From drill sergeants and squad leaders in the seventies talking about "gooks" and "slopes" to modern Crips who write all B's with a line through them, preparing people to fight and preparing them to be vicious involves a conscious cultivation of the enemy—or the victim pool—as "others."

2.2: asocial violence

Humans are nearly unique in the animal world. We are social creatures and so we have subconscious rules for social violence. We are also hunters and we know very well how to efficiently kill prey. We are primates, and do not rely on fang and claw, but on tools. We can juggle symbols and think of new possibilities.

We can use the tools and tactics that we developed to kill prey, tools and tactics designed to kill outside our species; and can use them to kill other humans.

A male lion will kill another male's cubs—but he won't hunt them. Leopards are quite capable of stalking and murdering competing leopards, but they don't. If a big horn ram really wanted the herd of females he could just blindside the other males from the side, crushing their ribs and knocking them off cliffs. But they don't.

Hunting our own is apparently a primate thing.

Not all humans can do this, and lots of research and writing has been done on the emotional cost to soldiers and cops when they take a human life. But this isn't about becoming a predator so much as recognizing one. You need to know that though most humans can't choose to ignore the humanity of their victims, some can. And those few, the predators, are an entirely different kettle of fish than any Monkey Dancer.

2.2.1: predator basics

Predators exist on a scale. Some few are pure predators, the classic sociopath. They do not sense any humanity, have no allegiance to the social contract. If a true predator wants your money, he has no more feeling for you than he does for the pocket you carry it in.

Most, however, are not that extreme. Some fake non-caring. Some fake caring. This is not nearly as important as you might think. No matter the level of anti-social you are dealing with, by the time you face a predator assault, one thing is clear: the predator has already decided that what he wants is more valuable than you. Do you follow? The Threat *may* have deep feelings for his fellow man, but if he is attacking, he's already gotten over them.

Predators do not see their victims as people, but as resources. Who you are has no more emotional weight than the wrapper his hamburger came in.

In a predator assault the Threat will use the tactics that he feels are the surest and safest way to get what he wants from you. He will take every advantage, relying on speed, surprise, ferocity, and weapons to

To explain a dynamic: Take a home invasion robbery team. The armed group storms into an occupied house and terrorizes the family until they are told where the valuables are. An individual doing this is likely a Process Predator (see below). A group will have a social dynamic, which implies that they are probably not complete sociopaths. It is possible that they will indulge in a Group Monkey Dance, especially if a higher level individual loses control or joins in another's loss of control. This is called a feeding frenzy. However, they are criminals and have imperfect trust in each other. If one begins killing, the others automatically have leverage when and if they are arrested. They have a murderer to give up. Killing is riskier for the perpetrator in a group situation than in a solo process predator situation.

try to cow you from responding in any way and to make any response you are able to access ineffective.

Predators are usually solitary. There are exceptions, but someone who sees others as resources has little reason to keep promises and rarely engenders trust in his own kind. It is not that predatory packs are ineffective or not scary, it is simply that they tend to turn on each other. Or become so suspicious that one will turn traitor, that they fall apart, sometimes violently.

2.2.2: two types

There are two basic types of predator. (See Fig. 2-002.) A Resource Predator wants something and has decided to get it from his victim. He is willing to use violence, but will often only threaten violence if he believes intimidation will work safely. The Resource Predator will use violence to get your money or car.

For the Process Predator the act of violence is the reason itself. The crime is the goal.

The rapist, the serial killer, ritualistic torture murderers are process predators. Muggings, car jacking and robberies are acts of a resource predator.

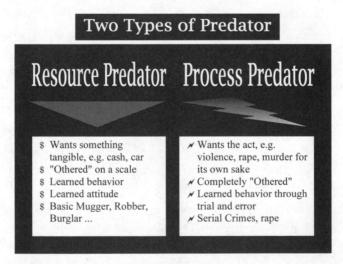

Fig. 2-002: Two Types of Anti-Social Predators

It is important to separate the types because the process and goals of the assault are different. Different assault dynamics require different ways to evade them.

The Process Predator requires time and privacy for what he intends to do. One of the reasons that home invasion crimes are so brutal is because our homes are set up to be secure and offer privacy. If the process predator does not come to the victim, he will try to move the victim to another place with more privacy and security. This is called a secondary crime scene. It is very, very bad. There is no good outcome from a violent criminal wanting to spend private time with you.

The fact that he is attempting to move you to a secondary crime scene or has invaded your home is a solid indicator that you are probably dealing with a process predator. If you do not end the situation it can and likely will escalate to rape, torture and murder. Any risk to escape is worth the price. Get out of there.

With a Resource Predator, you can usually give up the resource—your money, your car, whatever—and the situation is resolved. With the process predator, what you would have to give up is yourself. No deal.

2.2.3: two strategies

There are two basic strategies that either type of predator can use—charm and blitz.

The blitz strategy uses speed, power, and position to take control of the situation before the victim can make any resistance. Very important: it is not always physical. Many predators prefer to intimidate. If they can take psychological control, that's enough. A masked man shows his gun and screams, "Give me your money!" He is still using a blitz strategy even though the violence is only threatened. Psychological control, whether through simple fear or just leaving the victim with no good options but to comply, delivers his desired resource.

Intimidation is safer than violence when it works and it usually works quite well. In any act of violence, there is a possibility of injury. Things go wrong. Luck happens. Even the guy with all the advantages can slip and fall, or accidentally pick on the wrong cross-dressing martial artist.

Predators also are very aware of how the criminal justice system works. Far more resources will be dedicated to solving a crime with injuries than one where most of what is lost will be covered by insurance. If an arrest was made, the odds of prosecution and conviction are greater if the victim was injured. The potential prison time is much longer. In the first section, you got an overview of self-defense laws. Predatory criminals (and even low-level, non-violent criminals) for the most part have a good working knowledge of criminal law and the criminal justice system. It permeates the environment they live in.

In the charm strategy, the Threat uses his social skills to get the victim in a vulnerable position. A ruse as simple as asking for the time or a cigarette so that you look away for a second, or as elaborate as a pick-up artist seducing someone that he has no intention of letting live. Those are levels of depth—simple interaction to complex.

There are also levels of subtlety—"Hey little girl, want some candy?" is not as subtle as hanging around the playground appearing to look for a lost dog until a child volunteers to help. "Let's go back to my place" is not as subtle and rings more alarm bells than, "That looks heavy, let me get the door for you."

A skilled Charm Predator can set it up so that every step into his trap is one that the victim not only chooses, but thinks that he or she initiated.

When the Charm Predator has gained control, it will proceed like a blitz attack, especially with the intimidation option. The Charm Predator will generally gain control through location or position. If he has maneuvered the victim into a private place, such as his car out in the woods or her own home, he can then drop the charm and either go blitz with the immediate attack or intimidation: "I have a gun and your children are sleeping upstairs. If you scream, I will kill them."

In many cases, position is enough. If the predator judges that the victim is easily cowed he may simply display a weapon and escort her away from her friends.*

---

* Predators choose victims based on safety. Most predator assaults will be from men towards women or children, the most vulnerable target that offers the resource the predator seeks.

CHAPTER 3: AVOIDANCE

Rusafa Prison in Baghdad. Obviously, since I was here voluntarily, I'd failed to take my own advice on avoidance. Nothing immediately going wrong . . . how dangerous my immediate future would be, and how successful the mission would be could be affected by anything I did or said in the first minutes, hours or days.

So I asked questions like an inquisitive, well-behaved child:

"Why do men wear silver rings but women wear gold?"

"Why do some of the old men have dark circles on their foreheads?"

"Do you have pets at home?"

"What stories did you listen to as a child?"

"Teach me the numbers."

I found out very quickly that asking to be taught (out of curiosity, not out of a desire to control) is always received as profoundly respectful.

You have to understand violence dynamics before learning how to avoid violent situations. The things that might discourage a predator might trigger a Monkey Dance—you need to correctly read the situation you are in. You need to be able to recognize when you have crossed a border and are in a place with different rules in order to avoid the Educational Beat Down. You need to be able to distinguish between a Resource Predator and a Process Predator before you decide whether to give up what the predator wants.

There are three general strategies for not being assaulted: absence; escape and evasion (E&E); and de-escalation. If you are not in the place where the bad thing happens, you don't even get your feelings hurt. Absence is the most efficient survival strategy.

If you find yourself on dangerous ground, get the hell out. Escape and evasion is the first choice when you couldn't be absent. E&E

requires no contact with the threat, and thus, there is no chance of messing things up.

De-escalation is the last chance to avoid damage for both parties. There isn't always opportunity for it and it doesn't always work.

It is better to avoid than to run, better to run than to de-escalate, better to de-escalate than to fight, better to fight than to die.

Any option you take depends on your awareness, your ability to see confrontation coming. The earlier you see it, the more options you have. The more clearly you see it, the less likely you are to make a mistake.

In *Meditations on Violence* I wrote of five stages at which you can defend yourself from an assault. The first three of the stages mentioned—*blocking the motion*, *blocking the opportunity* and *blocking the intent* belong to the fight. *Altering the relationship* and *using terrain* are aspects of preventing the attack from happening in the first place. Altering the relationship is one tactic for de-escalation. E&E relies on a tactical understanding of terrain. Absence relies on a strategic understanding of terrain and crime dynamics.

3.1: absence

Bad things happen in predictable places. If you avoid those places you can avoid a huge percentage of the violence that occurs in the world. What are those places?

Bars, parties, and other places where people get their minds altered. Drugs and alcohol change the way people think and act. They lower inhibition and they make people stupid. When some of your brain cells are pickled or fried, picking fights can seem like a good idea. You may forget that "no" is a complete sentence. And that's just alcohol.

Stimulants can make people forget that they are mortal and can't really fight the whole bar. I have seen Threats on stimulants screaming and pleading and demanding for someone to come close enough to kill, so that, "We can all die together!"

High-volume cash businesses like bars and drugs attract armed robberies. Wired people with weapons can always go bad. People involved in the drug trade know that they have no legitimate place to turn to protect their business or make sure that agreements and contracts are honored. They have to enforce their own compliance and security. They are often armed and primed to use violence if they perceive a threat.

Note this: unless you are very familiar with that social strata, you will not know which of your behaviors might be seen as a threat or when you are breaking social rules. You must learn to recognize when you don't know what is going on *and keep your mouth shut.* More on that later.

Last note on drugs and alcohol, they do not only work on the threat. They work on you. If you need your wits about you to manage your own safety, stay away from intoxicants.

Anywhere that groups of young men gather is a hot spot for violence. The need to establish status and membership in groups drives a lot of the social violence. Young men are the most likely since older men, generally, have established their status and memberships. Older men still Monkey Dance sometimes, but it is more often power-plays at work than brawling in parking lots. Young men are more prone to violence. Young leaders are more likely to be insecure and use higher levels of force, to create a show. Last, a Group Monkey Dance requires a group. Avoid groups and you avoid the possibility of the Group Monkey Dance.

Violence also jumps off where territories are in dispute. Gangs fighting to control a lucrative drug market or an invading army both guarantee an escalation in violence. There is always some friction. Even when it seems that an organized crime group has complete

You will occasionally read apologists or even talk to survivors of totalitarian regimes who tout the order and peace of the regime. You might also hear old-timers talk about the safety of Mafia-protected areas in NYC and Boston. Monopolies on violence can bring something that looks like peace. As long as you obey. And look like the boss. And go to his church. Different types of peace have different prices.

control of a neighborhood, the cops are still working, good citizens are still resisting. It can make for a mentality on all sides that is more prone to violence than in a more stable environment.

War zones and gang territory have similar violence—including raids, ambushes and collateral damage of innocents. You do not have to be involved in order to get injured or killed.

Predators require privacy. They may lure the victim to a lonely place or find a victim there. A predator may charm his way into your home, the place that you go for safety and privacy. Murder, rape, and robbery are planned actions and they will occur in a place that benefits the attacker. That is part of his job, and an experienced predator is good at his job.

The more secure and secluded the place, the more time and privacy the predator has, the less he has to be concerned about your screams.

Predators vary in their dedication to the hunt. Most Resource Predators attack targets of opportunity. The predator wants something, so he goes looking for an easy way to get it. Or, someone who looks and acts too much like a victim comes into view and the predator thinks of what he would like to take.

Some like to stalk. They will haunt places, particularly places where people get their brains altered, and look for victims. The victim will then be hunted or lured to a nice, quiet place.

The next skill for absence is also the first skill for escape and evasion (E&E)—the ability to read terrain. Ambushes happen where you have limited mobility or escape routes, only one avenue of approach, and the Threat can safely get close enough to apply the type of force he intends to use. *Type* of force is not the same as *level*. In this instance it is about the range. An unarmed attacker or one with a knife must set things up so that he is very close. A sniper doesn't necessarily need to be in the same zip code.

Ambushes work best when you can be distracted—and not just attackers but pick pockets and purse-snatchers like victims who are focused on a good show or absorbed in window shopping, reading, and/or listening to recorded music. Anything that keeps the brain from sensing trouble.

The Threat will not always be hiding for an ambush. Watch how groups of young men stand at train platforms so that people have to walk close by them to get to the tickets or the doors. It is exciting for them to try to cause some fear, a way of counting coup and showing that they do have power.

If there is a place you must go and someone is standing in such a way as to force* you to walk close, there is a potential for an ambush. If the Threat is overtly intimidating, the danger falls on the social violence spectrum—make sure you have not invaded territory, do not look hostile or challenging. If the Threat is being casual and non-threatening, violence, if it does occur, will follow the asocial predator dynamic.

An assertive examination of the threat, not glaring in his eyes but scanning and noting his stance, possible weapons and where his hands are, will help to discourage the threat. He must see you scanning and evaluating. It sends a signal. Simultaneously, check yourself. Make sure your hands are free or any weapons you have are accessible. Scan for the Threat's possible confederates and keep the Threat in your peripheral vision. An experienced Threat will notice you doing this and will have to move you into a different class of potential victim, preferably out of the victim category altogether.

> Peripheral vision is vision from the side of the eye. It is not as focused as a direct gaze—you can't read with it and colors are less certain. It does, however, detect motion quicker and allow for faster response time than focused vision. A good fighter doesn't watch your hands, he puts his gaze where any movement from your hands or feet will register in his peripheral vision. The "thousand-yard stare" puts almost everything in peripheral vision and is a critical skill in combat to detect ambushes.

---

* He uses force in the same way a magician uses it. You have a choice, but what you will choose is pre-determined. You may *think* you are choosing, ". . . pick a card, any card . . . ," but the three-of-hearts will be under your hand when you reach.

Watch for ambush zones. For me, the easiest way to practice is not with the mind of the prey but the mind of a predator. There are too many variables in the world to notice every place where you are vulnerable. We are all vulnerable almost every place and at almost any time, if we don't use common sense. I'm writing this on five acres with three large, smart dogs between me and the only access road, but I am vulnerable to a Special Operations team that might have slogged through the rain and blackberries from another access road on the other side of the canyon. Yeah. That could happen.

So instead of looking at every place where you could be prey, start looking at the places you would set up if you were a predator. At what places on your daily route would you choose to wait for a mugging victim? If you were a Process Predator, of all the places you see in your day where would you set-up to make a quick snatch? How would a stranger get access to your home? You can play this all the way up to mass lethality situations (where would I come into the building on a shooting spree? Why that route?), and down to the simple (which car would I break into and why?).

The "why" question engages both your logic and your gut. It starts a dialogue between your instincts, which have evolved over millennia to keep you safe, and your intelligence. That dialogue makes both sharper. Trust your gut, but ask why.

Lastly—trust your instincts. Gavin DeBecker writes extensively about this in "*The Gift of Fear*," a book well-worth reading. You have an intuition that is always on, very reliable and only cares about you. When the hair on the back of your neck stands up or you get a very bad feeling, trust that feeling.*

Intuition is difficult to train because you never know when it works. If you get a bad feeling and avoid the ambush in the dark alley . . . nothing happens. In psychological parlance this is a negative

---

* Trust it in the wild. There are times, especially in training, where it is critical to face your fears. Outside of training you must distinguish between a touch of intuitive fear and simple dislike. If you followed the advice above strictly, you'd walk away from job interviews and tests. Know the difference.

(nothing happened) reward (and that's good). Negative reward, the absence of possible pain, is one of the slowest ways to teach.

You do know if it fails, however, but here's the problem. Intuition rarely fails. Not always (I do believe that most of the people killed by snipers never had any internal warning) but almost always, you *will* get an alarm bell. What fails is our response to the bell.

Force decisions are made in very little time and often, with very little information. Yet most decisions made by officers are very good. I use officers for this example partially because I have trained more of them but also because they are more likely to have had extensive experience in force situations. These decisions are largely intuitive and subconscious. Officers, write reports after-the-fact wherein they are required to point out what they saw and heard that caused them to make their decisions. Yet, intuition comes from the things you saw, heard, felt, and smelled that processed too fast for your conscious mind. The report-writing, done well, allows and forces the officer to consciously list the sensory details picked up by his subconscious.

As an exercise, I encourage rookie officers not to limit that practice to report writing—but that any time they get a twinge or a hunch they make time to track down exactly what caused it. This both enhances the officer's articulation skills (of why he did what he did) and also works that conscious/subconscious partnership, sharpening and strengthening both.

This is a powerful skill for avoiding conflict, and faster-than-conscious-thought decision-making will have a huge bearing on any self-defense situation. It will affect the legal and ethical decisions of Chapter 1 and the avoidance paradigms of this section. The ability to clearly explain decisions that were subconscious at the time will profoundly affect the legal consequences of the seventh section.

3.2: escape and evasion (e&e)

Not being there is always the best solution in self-defense. Avoiding the possibility, absence, is the first choice. If that failed or the situation was one of the exceedingly rare true ambushes or home invasions, escape and evasion (E&E) is your next choice after *not being there*.

The habit of studying terrain is critical here. You must develop a habit of knowing how to get out of places. Not just where the exits are, but take it to another level—what windows you can break, whether you can crash your way through drywall into another part of the building. You need to learn something about structures.

Until it becomes habit, notice everything you can about every building you enter—first, potential exits. Then, look for cameras, mirrors, shadows and reflective surfaces. In the buildings where you spend time, (your home, business, gym, or anyplace else) make a point of exploring them. Is there a basement? What is in there? Are the windows shatter-proof? How do they open? What is in the space above the ceiling? Are there passages above the drop-ceiling that cut through the load-bearing walls? Are those passages big enough for you? For your children?

The places you walk, the places you drive—do you take the same route? What other options do you have? At what places can you be cut off, forced into a dead space (privacy and time)? In any given moment in traffic do you have an opening front, back, right, or left in case you need to dodge and keep rolling? That doesn't always mean lanes. In Iraq, things like lanes and dividers and speed limits and even real roads were more suggestions than boundaries when under threat.

This is one of the big things about survival: when things are normal, you color inside the lines. When danger presents, you have to be able to break your normal rules and habits. Adults rarely run. At most, they jog. You have to be ready to run. You have trained your whole life to be polite. You will probably need to be rude. You enter buildings through doors. You must be ready to leave buildings through windows or over roofs or even through walls.

This book is focused on self-defense, but this is another skill with very, very wide applicability. You are far more likely to need your *safety bubble* driving because of an idiot talking on his cell phone than because of a kidnapping attempt. When you look at route-planning for ambushes you can also think about flood evacuation routes. Scouting for alternate routes will help you get to know your city better. There is no downside to this skill.

There are two critical elements to running away: do it safely and do it toward safety.

If you have already been targeted, running *will* draw attention. If there are guns it will likely draw fire. Without guns it can trigger a chase response. These are important to know but if running is the decision you make, run. Do not hesitate. Never, in a self-defense situation do anything half-assed. If you are going to run or hide or bluff or fight, do it with your whole heart. Hesitation is failure.

Running safely is using cover and concealment. If the Threats lose sight of you (concealment) they will have far more difficulty shooting you. Some chasers will also lose interest when they lose visual contact.

Cover is anything solid enough that it can stop whatever the bad guys are shooting at you. Try to keep cover between you and the Threat. And be sure you know the difference between cover and concealment. The walls in most buildings are not cover. Even a handgun bullet will go right through them. We were told when learning building searches that our partner's armor was the only decent cover in a stick-built house.

Distance can work for both cover and concealment. Even trained officers miss most of the time at extremely short ranges. Be a moving target and get distance.

If you get injured—shot or otherwise—while running, keep running. Most people survive wounds. Most wounds are psychological, not physically incapacitating. You may be killed. You may bleed-out. DO NOT give up. Not even if you are shot.

"Run towards safety," says Michael Jerome Johnson, martial artist and fight director of stage and screen. The instinct is to run away from danger. That can be blind, because you are more focused on the Threat behind you than on where you are going. Adrenaline—hormonal fear—can make you clumsy and limit your vision. You need your focus on your route and your own feet.

You will be afraid when you run. That is why you are running, so it is okay. But you must run smart and staying smart is very hard to do when you are scared. There is a concern that you must be aware of—running can put you in a panic mode. Fear breeds fear. Panic is unacceptable. These are just words and words rarely help, but here is the advice: You avoid panic by staying focused on what you are doing. Not on how you are feeling about it; not on what might happen. Focus on what you are doing.

One other piece of advice that works for me, especially in the fight: make a conscious effort to smell. Something about keying into scent not only assures that you are breathing but also helps bring you closer to your predator mind.

In running towards safety remember that if you walk into a situation, like an armed robbery, the route you took in is likely still safe for leaving.

A chase, if it happens, will not be a Hollywood fantasy of empty alleys. And chases are actually pretty rare in the woods. If no one is around, there's nobody to chase you. In most cases in the industrialized world running to a large group of potential witnesses is also a very safe bet. Run towards light and towards people.

"The Superior Man uses his Superior Judgment to avoid using his Superior Reflexes."

If you can't be absent, run early and run often.

3.3: de-escalation

In Section 3.1, we talked about avoiding places where conflict was likely. 3.2 was about escaping from places where conflict was imminent. 3.3 will be more personal. There will be times when the Threat has made contact or you have become aware of him when your last option, before it goes bad, is to convince the Threat to take another way.

Like medicine, the cure must be based on the diagnosis. A bacterial fever is treated differently than a viral fever. De-escalating a Monkey Dance is not the same as de-escalating a Charm Predator. You must understand and be able to recognize the different types of violence in Section 2 in order to have a chance at de-escalation.

3.3.1: know thyself

You already got a start with examining some of your inner workings in 1.2. How you de-escalate will be greatly influenced by who you are and how you present yourself. Physical counter-intimidation won't work unless you have a physical presence. That doesn't mean you have to be big or cut, but if you look ill-at-ease in your body, awkward and uncoordinated, it will be hard for a potential Threat to take you seriously no matter how big you are.

You need to study your own face. You can't see your own face or hear your own voice under stress. Everyone reads body language and facial expressions all the time, but yours probably tells more about yourself than you want to give away. Conversely, when you consciously try to send a message with a look it may not convey what you wish.

After discussing this with my jujutsu students one showed me his attempt at an intimidating stare. It looked like a ten-year-old trying not to cry. Rookie team leaders often have their voices squeak from adrenaline the first time they try to talk a barricaded Threat into surrendering. These are not things you can learn by guessing. You have to step outside your body to see how you look and sound.

Record your own voice. Watch your body language in mirrors and video. See how others see you, especially when you are trying to get them to do something. The insight of seeing yourself from the outside is invaluable.

What follows in the rest of the chapter will be heavy on techniques that have worked for me. But, you are not me. I'll try to present the underlying principles that made my stuff work. Use the principles to create your own stuff, tactics that are in keeping with your nature.

Remember, also, that my stuff doesn't work all the time. Once upon a time I was staring down 190 inmates about to riot. I'd tried reason, rejected trying intimidation (there were too many for any threat I made to be real, it would have just set a match to the gasoline) and had pretty much decided to sell my life for as much damage as I could when I was saved by Kari, an older female officer.

"Well, I never. I'm ashamed of you. I have kids of my own and I have never heard so much whining in my life and you're supposed to be grown men." She had her hands on her hips and a pursed-lipped look of scolding disappointment. Kari mothered us out of a riot. She's my hero.

There are certain lifestyle changes that can make you less likely to be a victim and at the same time increase your options for dealing with violence. Lifestyle changes are big. We have all observed how hard it is for some to quit smoking or lose weight. But the big changes have massive impact across many areas of your life. Only you can decide if it is worth the effort and if you have the discipline.

Get in shape. It makes you look less like a victim, plus it also makes life more fun. Your own body is the best toy you will ever have. It's more fun tuned-up. That said, I'm not talking necessarily size or strength, or looking good. For both self-defense and fun, work for agility and grace—moving efficiently. Train in something that makes it a joy to move.

Pay attention. A lot has been made of the Cooper Color Codes—putting yourself on red alert when danger is imminent—stuff like that. The thing is that the skill to see and identify a Threat is exactly the same skill that makes walking down the sidewalk a fun adventure in people watching and geology and architecture. You live more fully, and that is even more of a benefit than the fact that predators will read you as a harder victim.

Learn all you can. Whether it is Musashi's advice to "become acquainted with every art" and "know the ways of all professions," or another path, the more you learn, the more you can understand. The more you can understand, the more people you can reach and outcomes you can affect.

Don't mess with your brain chemistry. Your brain is a finely balanced machine. You can usually make it stupider with chemicals, not smarter. Don't be dumb on purpose.

Get to know the guys on the ground. Make a habit of getting to know the support staff where you work, the cleaners and security officers and maintenance team. Even children will know and share things that others miss.

Consider these efforts an investment in your safety.

That's the point, mothering is not a tactic that would work for me. Don't limit yourself to what I present.

3.3.2: know the world you are in

There are lots of different worlds. After spending fifteen years working the jail I was rotated to an office job as an investigator. I got along well with officers and inmates, but headquarters was an alien environment. I did not understand the core beliefs shared by my fellow cubicle rats, and thus could not, at first, understand their values or respect their etiquette. Worse, I didn't realize for some time how different their values were, and how nervous I made them. Live and learn.

Jail is different than office is different than home is different than the gym or dojo. Keep your radar active whenever you find yourself in an unfamiliar place. Your intuition should give you a little warning bell when you are out of place. Trust it, and then look around. Most of the things that trigger it will be groups who stand at a different distance than you do (different ideas of personal space) who maintain eye contact differently (inmates and ex-cons have a tendency to avoid direct eye contact and instead look over each other's shoulder, mutually looking for danger) and who talk in different tones (some cultures are very loud when they are not angry; other cultures are very quiet, which can feel like everyone is whispering secrets).

Blending-in is less a matter of imitating these behaviors, than showing comfort with them. Try to be slightly lower on the scale, more invisible, than what you see around you. Don't freak when someone invades your space, (unless he is doing it much closer than the locals do with each other) but don't invade another's space. Talk just a little lower than everyone else. Make slightly less eye contact than you see around you.

Eye contact is a tricky one. Direct eye contact can be required to show respect or be taken as a challenge depending on culture. Evading eye contact can be taken as deference or deception. My usual tactic when talking with someone who may be or become a Threat is to focus on the mouth. Looking at the mouth in direct conversation shows full attention without triggering a challenge.

To scan a room, look at each person, scan the interesting ones up and down once, and move on. Do not hold eye contact. When you move on to the next person, break eye contact sideways, not up (can look snobby or dismissive) and not down (which will look submissive). Unless you detect an immediate, overt threat (like a gun—think Means rather than Intent) move on to the next interesting person after a scan. This shows alertness, some skill and *no challenge*. In the peaceful world, most won't notice you scanning. If you have stepped through the looking glass into a more conflict-prone area, those that do notice will see it as a sign that you know what you are doing. Do not lock eyes during a scan if you want to avoid conflict. If someone is staring at you, look back, possibly nod, and steadily move your gaze to someone else. Act as if you see no challenge whatsoever in the stare.

When scanning, look for interesting body language. Trust your gut first and foremost. The ones that naturally draw your attention deserve the single scan. If it is a woman do not scan any slower and for god's sake do not lick your lips. Just sayin'.

Other things to look for during the scan include who is carrying weapons (concealed or overt, types of weapons) whether the clothing is designed to conceal weaponry, such as hanging shirt tails or loose open front shirts over t-shirts and whether weapons or the possibility of weapons are the norm or the exception.

This is especially important for women: during the scan note if women are there without a male escort. Subcultures with propensities for solving problems with physical violence usually have very strict rules about how men and women act and interact.

There are some places where a woman may only go with her husband, others where she must have a female escort and some places where unescorted women are assumed to be there for paid sex. If you are an unescorted woman in one of those places, leave. It helps to look and act embarrassed to have made a mistake.

Please, for your own safety, do not stand on some misguided idea of the way the world should be and deny that these places exist or that you have entered one. Denial of reality based on high-minded (but naïve) principles can carry a very high price.

Borrow intuition cross gender as well. There are a number of men who give almost all women a "creepy vibe" but don't trigger a reaction from men. If you are a woman, trust the vibe. If you are a man, notice the signs in the women around you (when the guy wants to hug as a greeting, women pull away; women use greater distancing and tend to stay with other women when the guy is around . . .), then:

1) Keep him on your radar; and

2) Don't leave women alone with him.

Borrow intuition. You can usually assume that most of the people in any given place spend some time there and know the rules and the power structure. If everyone looks up and checks their weapons when a certain person walks into the room or stands, congratulations. You've just identified a dangerous guy. If most people are comfortable standing very close but leave a wide space around one table, those are probably the players. If the patrons of a bar are lewd and rude to all the girls but one, you know who the boss likes. You can get the lay of the land by watching the natives.

When you are or believe yourself to be on dangerous and alien ground, keep your mouth shut. This is hard for some people. I can't help but think that if you don't have the common sense to keep your mouth shut or you believe that your opinions and insight are so precious that everyone wants to hear them, then you probably will suck

I don't give a damn about your self-esteem. The purpose of this book is to give you a few hints on staying alive or, if you teach self-defense, some critical information you can pass on to your students. The world is not about you. Everything that you know about right and wrong is context dependent. If you go to a place that is outside your context and demand that they treat you by *your* rules in *their* world, not only might you get killed, but you will be killed for being a whiny child demanding special treatment. If this is you, its time to grow up.

at avoiding conflict anyway. Get this, the commanding presence and facile vocabulary that made you president of your college debating team will be triggers that can get you stabbed or beaten in a different social environment. The charm and over-the-top personality that made you prom queen can get you gang-raped.

You must recognize when you are an outsider and know that an outsider drawing attention rarely ends well.

If you find that you have stepped into a danger zone, do you need to stay there? If not, leave. Quietly. Politely. If you have already entered and sat down (which implies you weren't paying attention earlier in the book) order one beer, leave a nice tip and go. You came without friends, leave without friends.

If you came in with friends, particularly a woman and you are worried about her safety, leave now. Don't waste time. And do not spend time, ever, with women who feel it is hot for you to fight for them. No matter how good the sex is.

If you get addressed or called into a conversation, be polite. Polite is not the same as meek or timid. Those can draw attention to the fact that you don't belong there. The less tension you show, the less sure anyone will be that it is safe to push you. Say as little as possible. Listen. The more you talk, the more likely you are to give away a hook (see later). When violence goes down from this situation it can break as a Group Monkey Dance, a Monkey Dance, a Status Seeking Show, or you can earn yourself an Educational Beat-Down.

If a Monkey Dance starts to kick off on dangerous ground, look at the audience, shake your head, show your hands, palms out, and leave without saying a word. It satisfies the Monkey Dancer, gets you out of there, no one is hurt and you have not said anything that could make it personal and escalate it to a Status Seeking Show (SSS) or Educational Beat Down (EBD).

If you find your way blocked, the situation was pre-set for a Group Monkey Dance (GMD). The receiving end of a GMD is one of the worst places you can be. Explosively break through the block, and run out of there. If you move fast and decisively you will be able to knock down or push past almost anyone.* If you try to stand and make it some kind of contest, the others will be on you very quickly. Too quickly.

If a GMD is starting (e.g., there is no single person Monkey Dancing with you but several are trying to surround, intimidate, or cut off your exits) it will be very, very bad. If it is a low-level GMD (just letting the outsider know he is not welcome) they will often tell you exactly what you need to do to get out unhurt: "Son, you get out right now or we are going to kick your ass."

That is a whole conversation. It is an if-then statement. Just do it. Your little monkey mind will want to throw out some kind of face-saving gesture, to negotiate or argue or show a glimmer of defiance, to set some terms. "Okay, I'll leave as soon as I finish my beer."

That comes from the little monkey in your head who wants to be an alpha male and have a whole harem of fine chimpanzee females. That little monkey in your head is stupid and will get you killed. If someone tells you what you need to do to get out alive, do it. And keep you mouth shut. Unless part of the instructions were to apologize. Then just apologize, no weasel words, and get out of there.

---

* This needs to be practiced. Many students trying to crash a blocked path will run up to the opponent, come to a full stop, set, and then try to apply power. The success of this technique is in *not* stopping—crashing right through.

You probably feel vaguely superior right now. It's nice to be civilized enough that you only have to worry about situations like this if you accidentally get stuck with some less evolved primates.

That's exactly the attitude that they will sense and will result in your beating. I don't care whether it is a watering hole in a coal-mining town or a jail or on the "res," you have nothing to feel superior about. These men and women have survived under these conditions and these rules for a lifetime whereas you might not survive an evening. There are things we can prefer, but nothing to feel superior about, especially when projecting that feeling can get you killed. Dead is the ultimate in inferior.

This happens a lot and I never noticed until Marc MacYoung pointed it out. Lots of **social violence comes with instructions,** and ignoring those instructions automatically puts it in the Educational Beat Down (EBD) category. If the instructions are ignored with arrogance, the EBD will be a show and it will not be good.

When an EBD is in the offing, unless you have done something outrageous, a sincere apology goes a long way. Outrageous is different in different places. Touching the boss' girlfriend is almost always on the list, though.

Watch carefully to see that the EBD does not escalate:

Threat: Hey! You can't just grab the phone we're all waiting. (points to several men in near-by chairs)

Fish*: Sorry. I didn't realize there was a line.

From here, it can break several ways. If the Fish lets his monkey-brain do the talking, he might try to negotiate:

Fish: I already started dialing, let me finish this phone call, okay?

In many cultures with a propensity for violence there are very strict rules about how men and women interact. Unless you know the culture very well, assume that members of the opposite sex are off-limits. If you are a man and a woman approaches, be polite, reserved, and respectful. No contact, no excessive eye contact. In some places, "Do you have family here? I'd like to meet them," will change the dynamic from a trap to a friendship.

If you are a woman approached by a man, ask for directions or something that would explain why a lone female (or all-female group) would be in a place where that was inappropriate and then leave. Asking for help, like directions, flatters the ego, gives an acceptable explanation, and usually prevents escalation.

If he offers to be your escort, "I'm not that type of girl" or "I'm so sorry, that wouldn't be appropriate, I shouldn't even be here. Maybe we'll see each other at . . . (fill in here, but Mass is always good in Catholic countries)."

---

* Fish is slang for a new inmate in jail or prison.

Threat: No, it's not okay. What made you special?

If the Fish backs down, no problem. He won't *want* to back down, but he did break a rule. If he doesn't or tries to salvage his ego with an insult or a dismissive look, he will probably receive an EBD. If you watch a situation like this develop, both parties will be throwing glances at the other inmates, gauging that they have support. The Fish won't have support, but if he sees other inmates gathering around and nodding to the Threat, the Fish had better back down. However if the Fish sees the audience giving the Threat a cold stare, this is less about education and more about a low-status member of the pack trying to earn some points.

In that case, the Threat, and the Fish, might escalate the situation into a pure Monkey Dance.

If the Threat is extremely insecure, especially if he is new to the group and itching to make a reputation, he may not let the Fish say another word. He may just explode into a Status Seeking Show, so that the audience knows that he is not someone to be trifled with.

The SSS doesn't have a lot of weight with old cons. They recognize the insecurity that drives it and can tell how the Threat picks out easy victims. SSS really only gets a lot of play with other young and inexperienced thugs.

So, there are four ways this scenario can end:

1) Fish apologizes and walks away. Essentially the Threat postured, presented himself as champion of the local rules. The Fish recognized that he broke a rule and now knows better. No harm, no foul, no injury and a little learning.

2) Fish doesn't apologize and it escalates into an EBD. This is most likely if the Threat is on the high or medium level of the social strata. That status, as well as support for his actions, can be read in the body language of the audience.

3) Either the Fish doesn't apologize or the apology is not accepted and things escalate into a MD. This will happen if the Threat is a low-level member of the social order (upper levels will not feel challenged by a fish) and he doesn't have the reputation for his attempt to enforce the rules to be sanctioned by the group. The audience will supply some of the clues for this but the big clue

will be that the language will change from being about the rules to about each other. "That's not how we do it" will morph into "You're an asshole."

This can also happen if the Fish tries to make it personal: "You can't tell me what to do," or "Back off, bitch."

4) The whole thing was an excuse for a Status Seeking Show. The Fish's apology will not be accepted. The whole point of the conversation from this point on is for the Threat to provoke the Fish into saying something that the Threat can use to justify an attack. Honestly, in the Threat's mind it is still an EBD. The Threat will say, if questioned, that he was teaching the Fish a lesson. He will also say that the Fish's words (which he provoked the Fish to say) left him no choice, even if all the Fish said was, "Don't touch me."

Your exercise is to review the conversation above and the outcomes and figure out why a GMD wasn't one of the options. As you read, make sure you understand the dynamic of what happened and why.

With the exception that it rarely goes to physical violence you can see all of these behaviors in any office. The MD comes up with two junior members arguing over the right way to handle an account, with neither actually thinking about profit or the job but just angling to win the argument. The GMD when the whole office starts ostracizing and spreading rumors about a member who made a big mistake or broke office protocol. The EBD when someone is passed-over for promotion after speaking-out to people higher on the food chain. The SSS is the public chewing-out by an insecure boss (secure bosses, good bosses, do their chewing-out in private for the goal of correcting behavior; bad bosses chew-out in public for the purpose of showing their dominance).

It's all primate behavior. I can argue that the physical violence is more pure and honorable than the slightly more subtle civilized version, but you can make up your own mind.

I use jail as an example because this is where I have the most experience, where I have seen the most permutations play out. You can see this same dynamic almost anywhere—in redneck watering holes, on the streets. Even in the corporate world. Just in the corporate world they try to keep the beat-downs verbal. All of the humiliation, none of the visible bruising.

Everything in this section about dangerous ground is based on the assumption that you are just passing through—that you have accidentally stepped into the wrong bar in the wrong part of town and you have no intention of returning. If you are moving in, if this dangerous and alien ground is about to become your home, the tactics you need differ considerably and may not be appropriate in a book on self-defense.

3.3.3: know the threat

This is a lot of information so far. It may seem like too much to make quick decisions, and quick decisions are vital in self-defense. It is partially a matter of practice and largely a matter of taking things that you already knew at a deep level and bringing them to your conscious awareness. It's not as hard as it might seem just reading the words.

You must be able to distinguish between a social and an asocial Threat first.

The distinguishing characteristic will be the presence of an audience. There are special cases—I have seen a few people who were mentally ill and would MD with no one to watch. For that matter I have seen one schizophrenic go through all the steps of the Monkey Dance with himself in a mirror.

Generally, though, social violence requires a society. An audience. If someone tries to suck you into what appears to be a MD with no audience, suspect that this is a Predator. If it looks like a pure MD, I would suspect a special type of Process Predator, one who enjoys the process of beating people. If you get sucked in, the beating will be savage.

Just as the Predator doesn't understand or ignores the convention that a dominance fight is validated by an audience, he also chooses not to understand where it should stop. If you fall for this trap and lose (which is very likely) you may get yourself killed. Certainly, you can expect to be maimed, crippled, or deliberately disfigured (curbing is the process of putting the already beaten victim's mouth over a curb and then kicking the back of his head).

Another sign of asocial violence is if you don't fit the profile for a status dance. If you are a woman, a child, or very old and someone starts acting as if they are Monkey Dancing or invading your space, prepare for a Predator assault. It might be a Status-Seeking Show (where the Threat is trying to break the rules) or, if it resembles pack behavior, a Group Monkey Dance in the offing. All three of these circumstances are high-violence scenarios. They do not have the built-in stops of most social violence. Regardless of which version it is, it is bad. Do not try to avoid it with social skills.

The exception is the Charm Predator, who may well approach in a crowd—but he will be there by himself and he will try to talk you into going someplace private. In a bar or at a party, how do you tell a Charm Predator from someone just hitting on you? It's tough because the charm predator is mimicking that dynamic and he may be very, very good at it.

I wish there was some sure fire way to tell you which is which, but there isn't. Not all men that fall under the category of Charm Predator get up in the morning and check off a to-do list that includes "kidnap, rape, and kill a co-ed." Some "all-American boy" who gets a little drunk and decides not to take "no" for an answer is also a Process

This book and others like it, (e.g., Lawrence Kane and Kris Wilder's *Little Black Book of Violence**) are a start. Taking martial arts or self-defense classes are a start, but don't be deluded. An experienced predator damages people for a living (mugger) or for fun (rapist). He is likely far better prepared for you than you are for him. Do not get over-confident.

* Kane and Wilder.

Predator. Since these two criminals, and the guy who is a little shy and has been working himself up for weeks to ask you for a date all behave the same, it is difficult to tell which is which.

Absence, a conscious decision to avoid places where strangers hit on you; or avoidance (as in a solid personal policy of never going anywhere alone or outnumbered with people you do not know and trust) are the *safest* things to do. That advice may not be easy for a young woman in college who wants to have adventures and meet people.* There are other ways to do that with less potential for certain bad outcomes. The choice will be yours. So will the consequences.

In his book *The Gift of Fear,* Gavin de Becker listed behaviors identified with the Charm Predator.** I can't improve on that list and it would probably be a copyright violation to reproduce the entire thing here. To summarize, charm is a learned tactic. People are not born charming, it is something that they do to make you like or forgive them. When someone is being nice to you, ask yourself why? Did he offer help or did you ask for it? Is he acting like you have some old friendship or personal bond (e.g., "Maybe we should do something about that")? Where the hell did this "we" come from? Does he ignore your protests? Make promises you haven't asked for?

These are also the tactics that salesmen use. And hostage negotiators. I have used them to develop rapport with inmates in an attempt to prevent the need to use force. Not only Predators try to be charming. Read DeBecker's book.

> Predators use charm to gain access, but they also use it to gain information. Something as innocuous as telling the handsome stranger at the library which dorm you live in might give him everything he needs to choose an ambush site. Be wary about giving information. Be especially wary if someone asks for information that they have no need or right to know.

---

* Most of my predator advice will be aimed at women, as they are far more likely to be the victims of predators. Most of the social violence advice will be aimed at men, for the same reason.
** *Gavin de Becker.*

Verbal de-escalation is ineffective with a Predator. With a Charm Predator who is trying to get you to go with him, a loud aggressive "I said NO! Leave me alone!" will usually work. Not because he will be put off by it. He doesn't care and it may even make him angry. It works because it draws attention. Predators do not do well with attention, anymore than cockroaches thrive in sudden light.

Most of the other common attempts to verbally de-escalate with a Predator are doomed to failure. Bargaining and pleading will probably backfire, simply increasing the Threat's sense of excitement. Predators in the wild will run *toward* the squealing of a distressed animal, not away. Bluffing and threatening will only work if the Threat believes you can back them up. Often, it will just give the Threat the hook he needs to rationalize what he wanted to do anyway: "Thought he could punk me out? I stomped him down *and* took his cash. He'll remember *that.*"

The Predator has already "othered" you to a sufficient extent that any communication that relies on a shared feeling of humanity will be ineffective. The Threat does not see you as the same species. Many of the social defenses to someone being a bully rely on an audience— being sarcastic or funny in the face of a physical Threat is intended to get the other people around you on your side and use peer pressure to make the bully back down. There's no audience when a Predator attacks, my friend.

Anything that makes the Predator feel more important or raises his self-esteem, like flattery ("You're really handsome; you don't have to rape."), or appeasement ("I'll do whatever you want just please don't . . .") can *increase* his level of violence. This is the soul of the looking glass problem: flattery and appeasement are common and effective ways to stop your boss from yelling at you or keeping him or her in a good mood. That is monkey social stuff. The stuff that works in social conflict backfires in predatory violence.

"Othering" is a very important concept. The true sociopath is a rare thing. This is the individual who can go through life like it was a video game without any emotional attachment whatsoever. They do not feel caring, tenderness, or love and cannot understand the concept that they should feel bad for breaking a heart. They feel no hesitation in taking a life and do not understand the concept of remorse. These specimens are, fortunately, very rare.

Humans, however, are almost always on some kind of scale. We divide the worlds by layers of connection. Watching a friend or family member murdered will affect you more than watching footage of 9/11. The 2,751 deaths at the World Trade Center will affect you more than the 273,000 who died in the 2005 Indonesian tsunami. The Indonesian deaths will affect you more than the millions of cattle slaughtered every year and the slaughtered cattle will affect you more than the billons or trillions of living plants that the cattle ate.

The most common hierarchy is: self, family, tribe (or friends), nation, species, cute fuzzy animals, boring animals, plants, germs, *scary animals*. The farther down this scale the easier and less traumatic it is to kill, for most people.[*]

Scary animals are a special case and it speaks to capacity versus capability. Most people will spray disinfectant or pull a weed without blinking an eye and possibly the majority of those people would never have the courage or the inclination to go after a man-eating tiger or shark. In that sense the tiger or shark falls in the usual animal level but with an *additional hesitation* due to fear. However, if a man-eater shows up or a nest of poisonous spiders or snakes is found or "the killer bees are coming!" (if anyone remembers the 1970s) the public outcry moves them to the top of the list for *someone else* to kill.

This is an important thing, but well beyond the scope of this book—our personal capacity to kill is one thing; our capacity to demand someone else do the killing is another. And how we feel about it after the fact when we feel safe again is a third and separate thing. Officers are investigated, sometimes charged, and often sued by families for doing what the families begged them to do when the fear was fresh. A panicked 911 call: "He just keeps threatening to kill

---

[*] Clearly, given that family members kill family members more often and that crime is most common in the criminal's neighborhood, there must be more going on here. Part of it is statistical—spending far more time with your family than with your enemies, rarer things happen eventually. Part of it is social, I don't know about you, but only my family really knows how to irritate me.

everybody" has been followed by a $14,000,000 dollar lawsuit by the people who made the call. Something to consider.

Most predators are not pure sociopaths. On some level they do know that people are people, that they are real and feel pain. But people can manipulate their own feelings. They can emulate sociopaths. The necessary skill is "othering."

You choose to believe, you convince yourself, that the person you intend to harm is not a person, certainly not a member of your family or tribe. If they are just an animal it is easier to do something you would have difficulty doing to a human. You see this in language designed to hurt or designed to give the aggressor an excuse to escalate: "You're nothing to me!" "Bitch!" The power of the racial epithets is in this "othering," and the reason they are used freely within the group is because there is pride and solidarity in being a special "othered" group. It is affirming to talk about your special nature. It strengthens the team bonds. It is dangerous to allow others to talk of it, in their mouths it is the permission slip they will use to kill you and yours.

Criminals do this. Power groups do this. Militaries throughout history have created slang and names for enemies and caricatured

"Othering" is not a *necessary* skill for people who use violence, however, and this might be something of a mystery. I have been exposed to a fair amount of violence and have used force as a professional tool extensively. I don't "other" people—much. I also seem to have a lot less of the associated stresses than most people who do what I do. The people in the field that I respect the strongest also have these three things in common: willingness to go in and do the hard stuff immediately; healthy lives and personalities outside of work and; no need to see the Threat as an enemy.

That does not mean that I think criminals are just like everyone else. There are some profound differences in the way that they think and view the world. To ignore this would be to lie to myself or to choose to be blind.

But it doesn't mean that they are in some way less than me. They have managed to survive in their environment, just as I have in mine. Reverse our circumstances and I might well have died as them and they might well have excelled as me.

I can recognize who and what they are. I can't put a value judgment on it. That allows me to deal with their behavior while maintaining absolute respect for their humanity.

That's probably confusing. I believe absolutely, that what the men and women in uniform do needs to be done. I've known too many of the victims to believe otherwise.

If you envision society as a ship, you have to scrape the barnacles off periodically. You don't need to hate the barnacles to do that. It helps to love the ship a little.

pictures to make them easier to kill. And, they have found that it is harder to kill people that look like you than people who don't.[*] "Othering" is a vital skill for people who use violence.

"Othering" will be most apparent as a tactic in the Status Seeking Show, when the Threat is looking for an excuse in his own mind or for

[*] Maybe that is why civil wars are so brutal. Because it is felt as a betrayal, the harshest elements of the Group Monkey Dance come into play.

Alienation is not "othering." Alienation is the very common feeling, especially in teenagers, that they don't belong anywhere, that no one understands the true self: it is lonely and emotional and angst-ridden. It results in the sometimes desperate search for a group where they can belong. It is almost the opposite of "othering."

Alienation is all about *me*. "Othering" is all about *them*. Alienation is begging to be included. "Othering" is learning skills to exclude others.

the benefit of his audience to escalate to violence. If he is very success-ful, in other words if he gets you to say something that is an insult to his entire group, it can escalate to a GMD.

"Othering" is also vital in a Resource Predator assault when the predator wants to use violence but has no valid reason, e.g., you gave him your wallet but he still wants to hurt you, still wants the process.

Rationalizing is the process, after-the-fact, of explaining to your-self why what you did was the right thing to do. Maybe it was the only thing you could have done. Maybe even the noblest thing you could have done. Criminals are especially good at this. They have to be. It takes some pretty extreme mental gymnastics to be okay with sodom-izing an eighty-year-old woman.

Those are the pieces in the conversation leading up to a Status-Seeking Show, or the Predator who *believes* he is a Resource Preda-tor but *wants* to revel in the process—they are looking for what I call *hooks*—the excuses that will be used after the fact to rationalize the event.

There are a couple of things you need to be aware of here. First of all, these processes are subconscious. Predators don't think of them-selves as predators, much less process or resource predators. He wants something. He thinks it's money but he gets the money and he still wants something. What will fill the void?

The rationalization process is also subconscious, including look-ing for hooks in advance. The Threat has done this before. He knows, on some level, what makes him feel good or bad before and after the fact. He learned, probably as a child, that when he tells his buddies about the guy he pounded, they'll ask why and the story goes better with a reason.

Almost everything in the book is a subconscious process—not just for the Threat, but also for *you. You* get sucked into the MD. *You* freeze. *You* try to use boardroom tactics to avoid conflict in a violent bar. Hopefully in reading this, you will recognize it, bring it into your consciousness, and start using your conscious and unconscious mind to train each other.

Because it is now becoming conscious for you, and you are learn-ing to manipulate it a little, does not mean it is conscious for anyone else. The danger with understanding this consciously is that you may think it is okay to then discuss this and try to work it from the ethics level (see Section 1.2.1.1) when it is still a Belief/Values level problem for the Threat. You cannot communicate effectively at the conscious level with someone who is dealing with those issues subconsciously. You must bring them to consciousness (difficult and time consuming) or touch them at the subconscious level (which takes skill and a new way to think and see for most people).

I've written before (in *Meditations on Violence*) about the skill of not giving away hooks. This skill is simply refusing to be "othered." Arguing paints you as the antagonist, pleading as the supplicant. Threats believe they are reasonable, so you be reasonable back. Not condescending, not insincere:

"What you lookin'at?"

Maintaining extremely relaxed body language: "Huh? Sorry, didn't know I was staring. Just tired. How ya doin'?" There's no anger in that or fear or defensiveness. Even a little concern for your fellow man—"How you doing?" It is hard to "other."

No denial:

"What you lookin' at?"

"Nothing."

"Bullshit. You was staring right at me."

"No I wasn't!"

"You calling me a liar?"

Denial is a hook, it gives him an excuse to get angry. You are disagreeing. You must think he is stupid or a liar or you wouldn't disagree. That's all it takes to send things into a fight if someone wants to fight.

Being reasonable is not quite the same as being agreeable. I am not trying to make a friend or suck up—that can also be irritating and an excuse to escalate. The tone and tactic with a potential Threat is sincere but puzzled—if he won't let it go, you treat what he says—almost no matter what—as a thoughtful question and return thoughtful questions. Be careful, though, because if your ego, your monkey brain, gets involved you will throw out challenges while pretending you were being thoughtful.

"What you lookin' at?"

Maintaining extremely relaxed body language: "Huh? Sorry, didn't know I was staring. Just tired. How you doing?"

"You think just because you didn't get enough sleep that gives you the right to stare at anybody you want."

"Hmmm. Never really thought about it. Probably not a right, though. Maybe a pass. What do you think?"

If this drags out a little, it will be good. Most people require some adrenaline to fight and adrenaline burns out of the system relatively quickly. If you can keep someone talking calmly for a few minutes he will be far less likely to act violently unless he gets fired-up again.

There are opportunities for a few other tactics here. I've been very successful with bringing the emotions out on the surface.

"Partner, you sound angry and the edges of your lips have gone white. What's wrong?"

"You're bothering me, you prick."

Hard to keep your temper under a direct insult. The monkey part of your mind wants to MD. Keep it under control. "Mmmmmm, no. That doesn't sound right. It's something else." I'll even throw in, "Tell me about it." That's an advantage of being extremely avuncular.

If it escalates another step, I go one level deeper: "You're trying to make me angry. I just figured that out. How odd. Why do you want me angry?"

One that has worked a couple of times and is really funny involves a hurt tone and maybe even a quivering lip. "Hey! You're trying to hurt my feelings. How bad would you feel if you made me cry?"

Coming from a gruff jail guard this has completely shocked very dangerous men looking for an excuse to fight into absolute silence. Plus, it's funny.

There are two other verbal tactics that sometimes work when a Threat is building up to a Status Seeking Show. These may or may not help with a borderline Predator trying to give himself permission. If an audience is there, you can appeal to a member of the audience, preferably a female or a high-ranking male, "Ma'am, I really don't want to fight. I'm on parole right now. Can you talk to him?" The mechanism that you had to appeal to help (even more so for asking a woman for help) gives a boost to the Threat's ego.* If a woman intervenes, he can feel manly for not hitting her and allow her to pull him off or talk him down. This is less likely to work with the Predator because there is unlikely to be an audience and his goal is the pure hormonal rush of hurting another human and hearing him or her beg.

The second is the "little dog" or "the winner" tactic, in which you subtly explain why there is no status to be had in defeating you. Both require a certain physical presence, the little dog succeeds for the small and young. I used it accidentally when I was a teenager. The reason it works is because it is funny. I didn't know it was funny, I was just mad: "I'm not afraid of you. You think just because I'm little I'm afraid of you? Yeah?"** The Threat would feel like he was being challenged by a Chihuahua, and he would laugh.

*The Winner**** is a song by Bobby Bare. A legendary bar fighter, Tiger Man MacCool, is challenged by a tough guy (classic MD/SSS, the two blend). Tiger Man then explains to the beginner that he wishes him all success as a fighter while describing the injuries he himself had received from a lifetime of fighting. The prospect of fighting a legendary tough guy had a lot of ego pay-off. The prospect of fighting a one-eyed, toothless, partially deaf old man with a broken back,

---

Everything connects. Some things you should have been thinking about in Section 1.1: *Legal* and that will greatly affect the *Aftermath* (Section 7) will happen right here.

There are four elements in every fight: you; the threat(s); the environment; and luck. The law, in this day and age, is part of the environment and can affect the long-term outcome of any use of force. So are witnesses.

Attempting to de-escalate a threat or to defuse a critical situation are supremely important because talking someone down results in no

---

* If a lot of the process in social violence seems sexist to a modern mind, it is. These patterns evolved in a world of primate group survival. The world has changed. Our forebrains have changed. Our hindbrains, not so much-and fighting is largely a hindbrain thing.

** I didn't exceed 5-foot or a hundred pounds until my senior year in high school. Extremely late bloomer.

*** Bare, Bobby. *Lullabys, Legends and Lies.* Lyrics by Shel Silverstein. 1973.

> injuries and no lawsuits. It is as good as a win gets. It is also important
> because even when it fails, you are creating witnesses. It is critical for
> those witnesses to see and remember that you tried to leave, tried to be
> reasonable and did everything in your power to prevent the fight. If they
> remember that you tried, it becomes clearer—and this is critical for the
> civil suit—that the Threat left you absolutely no choice.
>
> Everything you say and do creates witnesses.

dislocated elbows and arthritic knees didn't have the same power or
bragging rights.

To repeat: de-escalation is *not* effective under a predatory assault.
If it wouldn't work on a bear (sweet reason, for instance) don't count
on it working on a human predator either. You can evade the Charm
Predator's system if you recognize it, but only in the pre-assault phase,
only before he cuts you from the herd. After that you have as much
chance of talking your way out as a rabbit has with a coyote.

When the opportunity is present (the SSS and the on-the-fence
predator have similar dynamics, so they were presented together) it
will be a very short window of opportunity. Once the violence starts,
it is too late to talk.

3.3.4: the interview

Talking is a social thing and it works better on social violence.
Conflict does not happen in a vacuum. It happens between people
and it tends to have a relationship behind it. Even in a pure predator
dynamic a relationship exists, if only in the Threat's head.

There is also a lead-up to the more social violence, in most cases.

The interview has become the common term for how criminals
get close to you and decide if you have the resource that the criminal
wants and how easily you will give it up.

For our purposes any verbal lead-up to a fight or assault will be
called an interview. The steps of the MD, already described, are one
sort of interview. The predator-on-the-fence or insecure male looking for hooks to justify a Status Seeking Show are other forms of

interview. The warnings prior to an EBD, described in Section 3.2 are yet another form.

The MD, GMD, and Resource/blitz Predator interview have yet to be discussed.

3.3.4.1: de-escalating the monkey dance

You should all be familiar with the steps of the Monkey Dance. Here it is, repeated, with options:

1) A hard, aggressive stare

Don't stare yourself. The scan mentioned in Section 3.2 gets you the same information without the stare. The thing with staring or even unfocused gazing is that the Threat will honestly believe that you started the whole thing. This belief makes it hard for him to back down. Staring even accidentally becomes a hook. The habit to cultivate is to watch people with your peripheral vision (which responds faster to motion than focused vision anyway) and pay more attention to hands than eyes.

2) A verbal challenge, e.g., "What you lookin' at?"
   Options:
   A) Treating everything as a reasonable question. *The tactic, described above, helps to avoid giving away hooks.*
   B) The Big Dog. *This is more of a mental game that you play with yourself. It can be hard not to be patronizing and you must not cross that line. However, if you can see yourself as significantly older and more mature, try to think how you would respond to this troubled young man if he were your son.*

   "What's your goal here, son?" I use "partner" if we're about the same age.

   "Wh . . . what do you mean?"

   "I mean that you sound angry and like you're trying to pick a fight. You don't know me, so it's not personal and you're too smart to pick a fight with a stranger . . . so, what are you doing? What's your goal here?" That acknowledges the issue directly, leaves no hooks unless you use "son" in a patronizing

manner, compliments his intelligence and offers him the subtle power of being your teacher.

C) Flipping the tables. *This is changing the rules of the MD completely. Best if used with humor because when the Threat recovers from his shock you want him laughing. Comedian Gabriel Iglesias, for instance, has an extremely effective high-pitched female voice with a giggle that would automatically defuse a Monkey Dance and leave the Threat laughing. Perfect win.*

D) Removing oneself from the dominance hierarchy. *MD is played with like members of the same group. Remove yourself from the group. This is a form of deliberately "othering" yourself and takes judgment. In certain circumstances it can trigger a GMD. Be careful.*

"Son, I'm off-duty and really don't need any paperwork tonight. Go fuck with someone else. Better yet, just finish your beer." In this one, I do use "son" (but never across racial lines—as that is seen as an attempt to "other" increases the power dynamic in my favor, and works against me in defusing). If you are not authorized to carry a badge, DO NOT CLAIM TO! This is also a tactic that can't be pulled off without a certain look. Remember, the judgment thing, this tactic could get you killed in a heavy narcotics trafficking environment.

Same tactic, different approach: back of one wrist on hip, other under chin, fatuous smile, "Oh, honey, I'm not a fighter, I'm a lover." This can trigger a GMD in certain circumstances and will be hard if the Threat has watched you for a while. This also has a limited window of opportunity. If you attempt this verbal after you have said anything else or, especially after contact, the Threat is likely to escalate it to a SSS.

E) Raising the stakes. *This is not the game that Marc MacYoung refers to as escalato, where each person in the Monkey Dance throws a little more ego in until they are too committed to leave. Nor is it the same as making such an egregious threat that it might scare off the other guy. Making a big threat can work to get the guy to back off, "I don't fight except to kill, little man, now go away unless you're ready to die." Remember you are creating witnesses and you have just made a statement where you brag about being a killer. This variation is a tactic that might help you at stage three but will ensure that you lose everything in the court proceedings at stage seven.*

Raising the stakes properly is not a challenge or a threat, merely stating that you have something too precious to lose for a game, "Partner, I'm on parole and I am not going back to prison for some little fight. Leave me alone." Saying "little fight" here is deliberate, implying that if you are going to prison whether you do no damage or a lot of damage, you might as well make it worth the time.

3) An approach, often with the signs of adrenalization including gross motor activity of arm swinging or chest bobbing, a change in color, usually with the skin flushing.

Gross motor activity, extreme flushing or pallor of skin, hands shaking, knuckles white, licking lips, are all signs of someone getting the chemical cocktail, a hormone dump of adrenaline and other stuff. From this point on, talking them down gets tough because they are no longer very good at listening. To be fair, if it got this far, you got caught up in the Monkey Dance yourself and if you are deep in the MD you won't remember anything I write here, but I have to try.

The first step to defuse at this point is to break eye contact. As a rule, you cannot talk someone down and stare someone down at the same time. Then show your palms and back away. Leave.

4) As the two square-off, there may be more verbals, and then one will make contact. It will usually be a two-handed push on the chest or an index finger to the chest. If it is an index finger to the nose (remember the face contact discussion, above) it will go immediately to #5. If there is no face contact, this step can be repeated many times until one of the dancers throws . . .

If you let it get this far, verbals are off the table. Break eye contact, show your palms and back away. Resist the urge to deliver some witty, face-saving insult. That is just your monkey brain trying to keep you in the contest. Defusing means leaving.

The pre-emptive strike (or pre-emptive act) is one of the surest ways to defuse a Monkey Dance. It is easy, safe and effective. If the Threat is on any level below four and you simply hit him or take him down his brain will be frozen. The MD, after all, is a genetic thing with specific steps. If you skip steps and he has to figure out what just happened, it buys you a freeze.

The problem is that the Monkey Dance is a two-player game. Whatever happens is mutual combat. You will not be able to claim self-defense and you have likely committed assault.

Some things that work tactically are suicide legally.

Cops can use pre-emptive force in a MD. Because they have a duty to act, they may not, by policy or law, be allowed to just leave. If they can tell that they will have to use force anyway, most officers can easily articulate why jumping steps in a MD allows them to take advantage of the Threat's freeze. That allows the officer to use a much lower level of force than he would need if he waited for the MD to progress to a fistfight.

5) A big, looping over-hand punch.

The fight is now on. You need to be moving, which means either fighting or leaving fast. Trying to talk, negotiate, or plan while a beating is coming in are not only ineffective efforts, but acts of denial. It is too late for prevention. Your goal now is extraction, getting out of there safely.

3.3.4.2: de-escalating the group monkey dance

Frankly, de-escalation rarely works worth a damn in a GMD. The attackers are into group bonding and almost anything you say will be interpreted as a further excuse to escalate the beating. Yell threats of vengeance? Just proof that you are an enemy. Plead? No one from *our* group would ever beg like *that*. Try to be reasonable? Too stupid to even know what is happening. Not like us.

There are a few things that work.

Acting crazy can work at almost any type of interview. Crazy people don't follow the steps of the Monkey Dance. They may not feel pain or fear so the Status Seeking Show can backfire. They won't understand what is going on and might not accept the beating, so the Educational Beat Down rarely gets used. Predators have plans and crazy can screw with their plans. Even the Group Monkey Dance, pack behavior wherein violence, weapons, surprise, and numbers can all be stacked toward the Threats' favor is riskier with a crazy victim.

Note well, there is a very particular kind of crazy that I'm talking about here. There are a lot of mental disorders that make people less aware and more passive. The mentally ill and emotionally disturbed are victimized far more often than they hurt others or turn the tables on an attacker.

The vibe you need to send is high-energy, paranoid-level alert, and unpredictable. You have to start in the early stages, which mean you need to recognize immediately when you are being targeted. Body language becomes jerky and rhythmic. Tardive Dyskinesia is the medical term for the side-effects of long-term use of anti-psychotics. Street people know the symptoms as the "Thorazine twitch." Sharp, small, rhythmic movements of the head from side to side. Twitching. The mouth is constantly dry so they lick their lips constantly in small, darting motions. If you have ever seen it, you won't forget it.

If you can fake these signs while holding a three-way conversation with Jesus and Elvis, people tend to leave you alone. Also, to any sudden movement (or no movement at all) suddenly snap towards it and stare with your whole body focused . . . then go back to what you were doing before as though nothing happened.

A lot of street level hustlers, particularly the homeless, fake this suite of symptoms for the same reasons as you might, to be left alone. We'll talk about de-escalating people in altered states of mind at the end of this section.

If you can get the group *laughing at you*, it may defuse the situation. It is not the wholesome laughter at a good joke, but the cruel laughter at something they find pathetic. This is the essence of the "little dog" tactic mentioned above. It is possible, in some circumstances and with some groups, to present oneself as too unimportant to be worth a Monkey Dance. If, however, there is a budding Process Predator in the group, they may want to play with you like cats play with mice.

The most successful way to stop a Group Monkey Dance is with an awesome display of force. You might get away with just displaying a gun if you have it, but be aware that if you ever display a weapon as a threat and the threat display fails, you will have to use the weapon. If you do not, it will be take away from you, and the person who did so will celebrate his or her own survival by dancing on your body.

A developing GMD is extremely, maybe unbelievably dangerous. I cannot give you advice on this, but for me, a GMD is the one situation where the risk of courts, lawsuits, and psychological consequences play little part in my decision-making because I know too much about the medical and physical consequences.

3.3.4.3: de-escalating the resource/blitz predator

Sometimes there is a pure ambush. Someone smashes you in the back of the head while you are waiting for a taxi or leaps out of the bushes when you didn't pay attention to the terrain. But the pure ambush is relatively rare. Even a Resource Predator who has no compunction about killing wants to get close enough to do it. Ideally he wants a little more.

The keys to de-escalating a Resource Predator interview lie in what the predator wants: proximity; a knowledge of you as a victim; distraction; and no witnesses.

Proximity: Be aware of anyone trying to get too close. You let people invade your personal space all the time. If a self-defense instructor says, "I never let people get within five feet of me," he is either deluded, a liar, or lives in a cave in the woods. People get close all the time. On buses and trains, walking city sidewalks at lunch time, waiting for a table in a restaurant—you have people within striking range almost every day.

What you need to notice are the patterns. Be alert to alarming patterns: Everybody crowds everybody in a busy bar, but people don't crowd at an ATM at night. If someone is trying to get close to you but keep you both distant from others, be suspicious. Most likely, you are being *isolated from the herd* where you will have less protection.

Don't hesitate to act. Tell the person to "back off." Make full eye contact with your hands up, but probably not fists. Use a firm, loud voice. Be rude.* This confrontation is a hard act for people who have trained their whole lives to be nice. Flush that. Be rude. Be loud. Be direct. At this point the monkey part of your mind will want to ensure you haven't hurt anyone's feelings, haven't damaged the good will of the tribe. However, people in your tribe, people socialized properly would not have violated your space.

Predators know the dynamic as well and they will try to use your social conditioning against you. "Hey, buddy what's your problem? Why are you being an ass?"

Lt. Warren Cook, long retired from the Multnomah County Sheriff's Office, once said that one of the most effective manipulations criminals use on officers is simply to say, "You aren't a very nice person." No matter whether this odd statement comes from a rapist, a killer, or a conman, the officer raised to be a good person consistently takes the statement to heart and does a quick analysis, questioning his or her own personality. This instant of self-doubt gives the criminal an edge.

Criminals use this tactic to sow doubt and it works, even on officers who should know better. If (when) a predator tries this on you, bull right through. He invaded your space. You owe him nothing. Not politeness, not an explanation. Just a simple statement. "Back off."

Stay on message. No explanations. "Back off." Many predators will respond with, "Or what?" Stay on message. No explanations. You monkey mind will really want to engage in a conversation to make sure all the monkeys around are mollified. The trouble is, this is not a monkey. This is a tiger and if you drop into monkey social behavior the tiger will eat you. Simply saying. "Back off!" must be *practiced*.

---

* Be rude-it is imperative for you to break out of the social monkey games. It does not mean that it is okay to antagonize. Antagonizing is another social monkey game. Be rude, don't be a dick.

The conversation part of your mind and the fighting part of your mind can't seem to work at the same time. I have done countless entries on inmates who were in their cells, some barricaded, some with weapons.* Whenever possible I make my move when they are talking. It takes all of them (so far) a short time to switch gears from talking (arguing, complaining or screaming insults) to fighting. This momentary freeze usually allows me to take them down and cuff them without injuring them. That's good.

As you can see, this tactic applied to the Monkey Dance will almost certainly backfire. But a version of this, the filibuster, sometimes works with the MD. That tactic is to go on a verbal tirade, accurate but never personally insulting, and keep it up until the Threat gives up and goes away:

"What you lookin' at?"

"Oh no, I know what you're trying to do! You say I'm staring but you know very well I wasn't so you're just saying that to try to get me to say something so that you'll say something so I say something back and it turns into a fight. Well not today. No way. Not today, not gonna happen. You just keep your staring and glaring cause I am not going to be suckered into a senseless fight, not by you, not by nobody. It just ain't gonna happen . . ." The Monkey Dance is an exchange: my stare, your stare. My insult, your insult. The filibuster tactic works on denying turns until the other regains his common sense and sees how silly the whole situation is.

Repeat: not all personalities can successfully use all the tactics I describe. And I'm sure there are millions of tactics I've missed. Life is a work in progress.

The second goal of a Predator's "interview" is *to gather information about you as a victim.*

---

* Remember IMO? Entering a locked cell gives the inmate opportunity. It is never done lightly. For officers, IMO includes Intent, Means, and Opportunity to disobey a lawful order. Many of my entries were on inmates who threatened or had harmed themselves, something for which Means and Opportunity are always present.

The first step will be testing how you control your space. If someone asks a question, how close do you let him get? And how, exactly do you send the signal that your space has been invaded?

If you pretend not to notice, especially if you try to shrink down and be small and inoffensive, you will make a pretty good victim. This is common and it is obvious where it comes from: being meek and silent prevents social violence. The message is, "I am not challenging you, I will do nothing bad, you do whatever you want and I will stay out of your way." This is exactly what a predator is looking for.

It is unfortunate, but humans can treat other humans as social rivals or as a prey species. There would be a lot less confusion on the subject of violence if predators looked like tigers and people playing dominance games looked like chimps. You are hard-wired to initially perceive a threat or danger signal from a human as a precursor to *social* violence, not predatory violence.

Very few will actually try to stop someone from violating their space. It's hard to do. Even self-defense instructors who say and teach, "Never let a stranger violate your five-foot circle," said nothing when I took the bar stool next to them after the seminar, or when a stranger sat on the other side. "Never" is a big word.

If you don't try to ignore someone entering your space, you acknowledge it in some way. That scan, when you look them up and down once? Very appropriate here. As is a non-committal, "Hi." During the scan, note whether hands are exposed or hidden and the possibility of weapons: bulges, clip-on knives, sheaths. Take a second to make sure your footing is good,* that you know in which directions you can move freely and that any potential improvised weapons, like a pen or a coffee cup, are close to hand.

It may sound as though the purpose of all this is to prepare for battle. That is secondary. The primary purpose is to send a message: *I see you. I have evaluated you. I am ready to go physical and I will continue to watch you.* The majority of people will not even notice

---

* Even if you are seated, move your feet into a position that gives you good contact with the ground and can launch your body, preferably in either of two directions, without shifting.

that you did this. Predators and people who deal with predators will. They will take it as a signal that whether the predator could take you or not, you will not make it easy.

Part of the signal is that you are allowing him to enter your space; you notice the breach of etiquette but display no intimidation.

Verbal protests, e.g., "This is my table," generally will be effective on a Predator if said with the right, serious tone (not loud or high-pitched which conveys fright). However, if it was not a Predator, it can almost certainly initiate a Monkey Dance:

"This is my table."

"Oh, yeah? I don't see a sign on it."

You can write the rest of that script yourself.

This comes up repeatedly: you must be able to distinguish a Predator approach from social violence because the defenses to one worsen the other.

A predator may often use a second, verbal technique to see how sincere you are. After you have given the scan and "Hi," or "That's my table" he could throw something out ranging from insulting ("Don't be a prick") to hurt ("I didn't expect you to be stuck-up like everyone else in this place"*) to ambiguous ("So?"). If you try to explain, or start a conversation . . . especially if you find yourself apologizing, you are still in victim territory. Tensions are somewhat high. Space has been invaded. It may have been invaded by a predator or by a monkey. By offering a conversation starter, the Threat knows that if you reduce the tension by engaging in conversation his camouflage is still intact and you see him as a monkey, not as the tiger he is. If *you* apologize, for *his* transgression he also knows that you are either afraid or believe yourself to have very low social status.

The Threat will also use his verbal and social skills to attempt to *distract* you. It can be as simple as asking for the time to get you to glance at your watch and away from the Threat, or asking for a light

---

* This one is huge. I have known several criminals who bragged about using this line: "I thought you weren't a stuck-up bitch like the others. I thought you could see beyond my . . . (past, tattoos, whatever)." Had the woman not fallen all over herself to show that she wasn't stuck-up and wasn't too good to be seen with the Threat, she may have escaped becoming his next victim.

or a smoke to both distract you and get one hand tied-up in your pocket, or as complex as asking for directions so that he can hit you while you are talking.

If you are already moving when approached, keep moving. Stopping when addressed by a stranger is a sign of deep social conditioning to be polite, or a submissive attitude to authority figures. Either reaction is blood in the water for a predator.

If you are already stopped (Review other aspects here. If the Threat is approaching you, remember terrain. Is someone moving to cut off your escape routes? Do you have cover you can reach or free areas to move through?), answer the question while keeping the Threat in full view. Avoid staring primarily because your reaction time to focused vision is slower than your reaction time to peripheral vision. In addition, staring may be taken as a challenge.

You may not be looking directly at the Threat, but you are not focusing your vision anywhere else, either. Show him your watch if he asks for the time (without holding your wrist out to him, he never really intended to look anyway). Tell him you don't smoke. If he asks for directions ask him, "How familiar with the city are you?" At no point give him an opening when you are distracted. The goal of de-escalating a predator is to make it too much work for him to bother. To some extent, many victims cooperate with their attackers by playing the social role that the predator desires.

Predators *don't want witnesses*. That's pretty obvious. One of the most powerful verbal deterrents is simply bringing attention to the situation before the Predator has successfully isolated you. There are relatively few completely deserted places and predators rarely hunt them because deserted places are not target-rich environments.* They must bully, herd, cajole, or order the victim to a secluded place for the real assault.

---

* Not surprisingly, hiking trails get a significant amount of violent crime. There are lots of solo and small-group hikers; generally unarmed; generally feeling safe in their environment; far from help; far from witnesses.

Bullying is using fear to make the victim comply: "You're getting in my car or I'll cut your face," or simply showing a weapon and taking her by the arm.

Herding is using fear and sometimes confederates to get someone to run to an unsafe place thinking, *there's a bad guy behind me and one up ahead so I'd better duck into this deserted dead-end alley.* Herding is intended to make you forget the cardinal rule that if you are going to run, run to someplace you know is safe.

Cajoling is what Charm Predators do only in a less sophisticated way: "C'mon, baby. Let's go for a ride. The city looks real pretty from up there on the butte."

Ordering, "You're leaving with me now" works sometimes. It shouldn't. Maybe it seems manly and some female soon-to-be-victims find that attractive. I suspect it is a conditioned response to authority figures.

In all examples, if the bad guy fears witnesses, your best protection is to supply them. Whatever you decide to say it should be loud, penetrating (shrill) and definite: "I'm NOT going with you! Let me go! Get your slimy hands off me!"

This verbal tactic is not an attempt to communicate with the Predator. At this point you are trying to draw the attention of all the non-predators around you. They don't need to intervene, often the attention and potential for witnesses and conviction is enough to get the Predator to decide you are not worth the effort.

Bullies choose their victims based on two criteria: safety and entertainment value. A kid who will fight even if he is going to lose, or one who has protective big brothers, are unlikely targets. It's not safe to bully them.

The kids who don't respond, don't scream or cry or show a response, those kids are rarely bullied. Just as babies like squeaky toys because it shows that they can influence their world, bullies like the power of causing an effect.

The preferred victim for bullying, then, is an emotionally expressive, physically timid person with no allies.

3.4: altered mental states

Pretty much by definition, dealing with a Threat in an altered mental state is a special case. The regular rules don't apply here, but there are several guidelines that have worked for me.

Altered mental states include the influence of drugs or alcohol, mental illness, and extreme emotion. The thing that makes these cases tricky is that what you know about dealing with people may or may not apply here. When I teach crisis communication to cops I go into a little detail about the different types of mental illness. It's nice to know, but it is not as important as you might think. If all schizophrenics acted alike and the way they acted was always different than autistics or guys on crack or people who are in a psychotic break, field diagnosis might be a more valuable skill.

Special case: no boundaries. This is something that is common with autism-spectrum disorders but I have seen a few cases with no other Autism signs. There are a handful of people who simply can't seem to read other people. They hold a handshake too long because they are waiting for an overt signal to stop, and they never notice that the other person is starting to get creeped-out. They stare at the wrong body parts. They are often too familiar, trying to hug or kiss hello when the relationship doesn't justify it.

You must set clear, definite boundaries. They don't see the boundaries, so they must be explained. Most will be grateful. If they try to argue or try to laugh off your boundary setting, expect a sexual predator who is already angling for the, "I didn't know I was doing anything wrong" rationalization.

3.4.1: rapport building

The most important thing is to recognize that the brain you are dealing with doesn't work like yours and you must be ready to adapt. Closely monitor what relaxes or agitates them and work with what you see. Here are some guidelines on establishing rapport.

Avoid direct eye contact. It makes those with autism spectrum disorder very uncomfortable and many in an altered mental state read it as a threat and can easily panic.

Listen. There are some who will go into the screaming/howling mode. If you can, get out of there. The howlers are a problem for people with Tasers and badges. If, however, a Threat in an altered mental state is talking, listen. Look for the internal logic in what he or she says. Let them know that you are listening and caring but *not* judging.

Don't directly challenge delusions. They hear the voices. They don't *think* they are hearing voices, they don't *imagine* they are hearing voices. They *hear* them. The same as you hear music or your friends talking.

Don't pretend to buy into the delusion either. Here's a news flash: most mentally ill people know that they are mentally ill. They have been dealing with it and coping with it for a very long time. They hear the voices and they know that no one else does. If you pretend to, they will know that you are a liar, untrustworthy, and patronizing. The specific tactic I use with delusional Threats is to say, "You know I can't see the blue men that you see. Let's try to concentrate on what we both can see."

Tie good behavior to favorable consequences: "No. You can't have friends if you're waving a knife around. You put the knife down and then we can be friends." And follow through. One of the terrifying things about being in an altered state of consciousness is the feeling of having no control. You can't control your brain. You can't trust your senses. Other people can lock you up or not. There is great power in showing a mentally ill person how to control parts of his or her own life. Even in a short interaction you can teach them, at least around you, that behaving nicely works on their behalf.

Unless they are being weird or angry, mimic their initial activity level. If someone is pacing, pace along with him. Talking rapidly? Start talking at the same speed. Keep at least one level quieter and less shrill though. Then, lower the volume of your voice and the speed of your activity and speech. Theirs will lower to match yours. You can sometimes calm them down just with this tactic alone.

When it is time for you to talk use a low-pitched voice. Dealing successfully with agitated people much less the mentally ill is very difficult for people with high-pitched voices.

Use positive (do) statements, in other words, tell them what they should be doing, not what they should not be doing. For example, say, "Let's walk on the sidewalk" instead of "Do not walk on the grass."

One of the things I tell officers is something you should know if you are in a position where you must try to talk-down someone in an altered mental state: "Have a second plan." Do not *depend* on anything to work. If the situation falls apart it can fall apart very quickly and violently. Be prepared at all times to use force if necessary.

My best tactic with mentally ill people and some drug users is to say, "When were you diagnosed (or did you start using)? Okay, so you've been dealing with this for X years. This isn't new to you. What should we do? What has worked before?" Being crazy doesn't require stupidity. They probably know better than you do what it will take to survive the situation. Ask and listen.

This approach probably won't work on people in a psychotic break and rarely works in excited delirium, two of the specific special cases.

3.4.2: the psychotic break

A psychotic break is when someone, usually with no history of mental illness, goes through the emotional wringer to the point that they lose touch with reality. This is the guy who takes his children hostage in order to demand that the courts give him custody. Or the guy who gets caught in a minor crime and escalates it to kidnapping and assault when he takes hostages trying to get away. Sometimes people get so depressed, angry or afraid that they will momentarily try things that are too stupid for them to consider in a normal state of mind. Cops call this a psychotic break.

Most of what is mentioned above will help but not asking them to solve their own problem. They simply have no more experience to draw on than you do. The two of you will have to work through it together.

3.4.3: excited delirium

Excited delirium is something that cops, Emergency Room doctors and coroners are entirely too familiar with. It usually presents as an enraged, frothing, naked man howling and growling and breaking glass, sometimes attacking anything he can reach. The nakedness is the man's reaction to a skyrocketing body temperature (liver temperature of 108F was recorded at one autopsy). I don't know why they break glass. They can be enormously strong and fast. My team dealt with one who pulled six concrete screws out of the wall with his fingers in order to break a stainless steel mirror to use as a weapon.

I don't know what causes it. Most are on stimulants, cocaine or meth or PCP, but not all. Most have a history of stimulant abuse but not all. Some have a history of mental illness, but not all. Most are fine when they finally get to sleep and wake up, except for whatever harm they did themselves smashing fists through glass. But not all. The 108-degree liver temperature was not survivable, I think.

Another, on whom we used a Taser to save, was never quite right but we don't know if it was brain damage he did to himself or the after-effects of an extremely high fever. I say the Taser saved him because he was driving his head into a wall full-force and the Taser was the only thing to stop him long enough that we could cuff him and get him to the ambulance.

Some in excited delirium die when they encounter the police, possibly shot, but sometimes they don't give up and fight until heart failure when the officers try to take them into custody without injuring them. I know an officer permanently injured in a fight wherein five officers were being thrown around by a single not-very-large Threat in excited delirium.

I have had nationally recognized experts tell me it is impossible to talk down a Threat in excited delirium. I've pulled it off twice. Both times I had very good back-up just out of sight and a quick escape route ready. I have no guarantee it would work for anyone else or if I could make it work again, but for posterity: I showed no fear (as far as I know). I entered slowly. I moved slowly. I talked in a low, slow voice. I told him everything I was going to do before I did it. "I'm going to touch your left arm with my hand. Good. Now I'm going to turn it a little and put handcuffs on."

It worked. Twice. Two successes do not make a system.

3.4.4: fakes

In Section 3.3.4.2 on de-escalating the Monkey Dance, I mentioned the value of being able to fake craziness and said this was a valuable skill among street hustlers. There are a couple of clues I look for when someone is acting crazy.

First, if a person's mental conditioning is getting out of control to the point that they become a threat, they are going to have trouble in other areas of their life, like hygiene. One of the early signs of someone in our mental health program starting to go downhill was if their hygiene deteriorated. You may not be able to see a change, in a street situation, but as a general rule if someone is clean with a well-brushed beard and hair and acting crazy, he is probably acting. Same with costumes. If someone is choosing clothes in order to make an emotional impression on strangers, it's a costume. One example was a guy in an urban college who carried his books in saddlebags over his shoulders.

If a guy is losing control of his mind, he won't take care to dress to impress. If someone puts on crazy clothes, that's a choice. If they then act crazy that's probably a choice as well.

The most important thing is a tip I got from the staff of the Oregon State Mental Hospital when we were transporting a very dangerous criminal to them for evaluation. I expressed my concern that the inmate was faking in order to try for an escape. The staff said, "It's usually easy to tell. Fakers try to act crazy. Real mentally ill people try to act normal."

Profound and dead true. Being mentally ill is no fun. Mentally ill people work their asses off to be as normal as possible and not let strangers know that they are different. They want to be treated like people and they work to earn that.

As a rule, if someone goes out of their way to let you know they are crazy, they probably aren't.

The last thing I look at is a simple test. Crazy people really don't have a choice. They can't just decide not to hear the voices or suddenly decide that their fear of enclosed places is irrational and get over it. Fakers can. If a guy is afraid to leave his room except when there is dessert, he's not that afraid.

We had a post where officers worked around both mentally ill inmates and mentally ill civilians. My officers had expressed concern because one of the private citizen patients, I'll call him P—was trying to stand too close and eyeing their equipment belts. I went up to check it out and immediately got suspicious. The guy was not only scrupulously clean but had a little costume going—he looked like a band member of ZZ Top with the big bushy beard and dark glasses at all times.

As soon as I got there and sent my officer out for lunch, P came over and tried to loom over me. "You got a gun?"

"Get away from me." I said. Level, low voice.

"You can't talk to me like that," P said.

"I'm not a nurse. I'll knock you on your ass. Leave." He left. Quickly, in case anyone thinks I was harsh talking to this poor, misunderstood mental patient . . . even if he wasn't faking he was asking about weapons and closing on officers. Sooner or later, unless he got shut down, he was going to put hands on an officer. With P's obsession with weapons, the officer might be in a deadly force situation. The officer would be hurt or killed and P almost certainly would be killed.

The whole point of verbal de-escalation is that you don't need to get physical. I would far rather be rude or cold than have to investigate a killing, especially one I could have prevented with a word or two. Even an ugly word.

3.5: hostage situations

There are different types of hostage situations and there will not always be a way to de-escalate. Sometimes de-escalation will not be up to you. If there is a professional CNT (Crisis Negotiation Team) involved, let them work their magic. There are some things you can do to decrease your chances of dying.

First and foremost, if a large body of armed people storm a place (school, theater, mall) run. Get out of there no matter what. Even if you are shot. The goal in a terrorist siege will be to capture a large group, put them in an easily defended place, *wire the hostages to explode*, and kill as many hostages, rescuers, cops, and reporters as possible. The surviving bad guys will then try to escape in the crowd, possibly posing as ambulance personnel or volunteers helping with the wounded.

They will maintain control of the group by killing or raping in front of all the other hostages anyone who shows resistance, leadership, or smarts. Comforting children, doing anything you might learn in a hostage survival class, or using anything I advise here will identify you as someone who has trained to survive and lead to your summary execution.

If you see one of these situations coming, run.

For most other potential hostage scenarios killing all the hostages does not serve the goals of the hostage taker. For irrational threats, the rapport-building advice from 3.4.1 will help. The advice for recognizing when you are on deadly ground will help. The standard advice for hostage survival is to *personalize* yourself and *minimize your differences* from the threat.

Personalizing yourself is to try to start conversations with the hostage takers where you present yourself as a good, genuine person with as much in common with the Threat as you can find. It is harder to kill someone you know than a stranger.

Cops taken hostage are often advised to minimize their differences by removing their uniform shirts as soon as they can find an excuse.

These should sound familiar. Here's the deal.

You must not let yourself be "othered." The more "other" that the bad guys can convince themselves you are, the easier it will be to use violence and the greater the violence they will feel comfortable using. Personalizing is an easier, more positive (do statement) way to say it, but the mechanism is "othering."

Some advice from Peyton Quinn:

Do not insult.

Do not challenge.

Do not deny it is happening.

Do leave the Threat a face-saving exit.

CHAPTER 4: COUNTER-AMBUSH

Talking to a friend in a public place, her eyes suddenly focused over my shoulder and went wide. I turned fast, elbow up, spinning and drop-stepping towards the Threat. Didn't feel the solid contact of a head, but felt an arm brush away and continued. The drop-step placed me behind the Threat and one hand came up to grab the face and control the spine, the other found a bendable wrist.

And I stopped. A friend playing a trick. Sigh.

Avoidance and de-escalation have failed or you never had a chance to use them. You have been attacked. Something just broke over the back of your head or someone has grabbed your hair and yanked you towards a closet. What should you do?

Let's take it back one step. What should you already have done before you even realized the fight was on?

This section covers only about a quarter of a second of any fight, but it is a crucial damn quarter-second.

I'm less worried about the Monkey Dance in this section. If you couldn't get out of that it's on you. Additionally, the MD is not particularly dangerous unless you fall and hit your head. This is about surviving the first contact of an assault in such a way that you can recover.[*]

4.1: foundation

What you need must be fast, effective, uncomplicated, work on most things without modification, easy to train and you must be able

---

[*] In case it is not clear, a fight is two people trying to hurt or physically dominate each other. An assault is a single person attempting to hurt or dominate a victim. If a victim of an assault can turn that into a fight it is a significantly improved situation.

to follow it up. Sound simple? Then, after you've got it you must train it to reflex speed.

Fast. Ideally, the move would be so efficient that upon your first clue of an incoming attack you could launch and hit first. Because reaction is slower than action this is hard. Not impossible, just hard. At minimum, when trained to reflexive speed, this move should be fast enough that if you are hit you will hurt the Threat before his second attack lands.

It must work. That's almost too obvious to say, but I have seen many moves taught that are not workable in real life or under real attack conditions (e.g., catching knives in the air, somehow getting your elbow between a fist and your face faster than the fist can move or wrist locking a fast flurry of punches).

Simple. If the move is complex; it will be too slow to employ, too hard to train, too easy to over-refine to the point of uselessness. Simple works better in the slop of real combat than complex.

Without modification. The move should work on most common attacks. If you have to change the move to accommodate where or how the attacker stands or whether he attacks with a right or left hand or high or low, it requires a series of decisions that slow you down. Thinking is too slow in a fight. You need an initial move that works on (almost) everything.

Easy to train. You want to put a lot of repetitions into this to make it reflexive. You also want to be able to practice it at full power and speed safely.

You must be able to follow it up. This is a reminder for *me*. I have a few counter-assault moves that I love, but I am an infighter. If you are not an infighter and use my entries, you will get past the first quarter second with flying colors . . . and then have no idea what to do.

Train to reflex speed. If you have to think, the Threat's second strike or the third will land. Every strike that gets in, every stab, decreases your physical ability to do anything about the next. Time is damage. Damaged is defenseless.

4.1.1: elements of speed

There are some concepts that will help you understand what speed is and how it works in combat. These are critical elements in Chapter 6: The Fight, but they come into play on a different level here.

The OODA loop, developed by U.S. Air Force Colonel John Boyd, is the standard model for decision-making in combat. All decisions occur this way. Until you train yourself to skip steps, that is.

O—Observe. First you have to see what is happening. If you don't see it coming, you can't do anything about it.

O—Orient. You don't get the information with commentary. You see a flash of something shiny coming at your belly. That's Observe. "Oh my god that's a knife!" and "He's stabbing me!!" are Orienting, figuring out what the "shiny" is. If you can't figure out what is happening, you can't do anything effective.

D—Decide. Only after you've Oriented can you decide what to do about it.

A—Act. You don't even begin to move until after the Decision is made.

If the Threat's Action, his punch or stab, is your first Observation, you begin the OODA process three steps behind the threat. It is hard to catch up. Every Action is something to Observe, so if the Threat's attacks come in faster than you can Orient and Decide you will keep recycling to the start of the loop and never Act. A flurry of attacks is one of the best ways to induce freezing in others. Professional bad guys know this.

This loop is also the basis for the maxim that "action beats reaction."

The slowest parts of the OODA loop are usually Orient and Decide. Your ability to Orient quickly is largely a product of training and experience. The more things you experience, the more closely your training matches real violence, the faster you will recognize bad things happening. If you recognize when a hand slipping to the waistband is a weapon check you know you are in an armed encounter.*

---

* People who carry concealed weapons have a habit of checking to make sure that the weapons are still there and haven't shifted. I draw the back of my thumb across my waistline. I am so used to being armed that I do it even when I'm not packing. It's still a clue.

With experience or training you can tell a weapon check from a draw and act accordingly.

Your ability to decide is based on many things. Surprisingly, if you are well-trained and have "lots of tools in your toolbox," that can slow you down as you waste time trying to select the best tool. You don't have time to waste when someone is trying to hurt you.

If you have an instinct to gather information before you make critical decisions, it can destroy you because in an assault much of the information you gather will be about what brutal things the Threat is

> As every martial artist knows, most strikes are telegraphed. The eyes focus, the breath catches, the shoulder drops or the hand goes back, all before any strike happens.
>
> Blocks are not telegraphed. If they were, they would be too slow to be useful. Remarkably, even when they are the same motion, the strike is telegraphed, the block is not. Meditate on that, and consider that your counterassault should be un-telegraphed and instinctive, like a block. Even if it does damage like a strike. (See Figs. 4-001 and 4-002.)

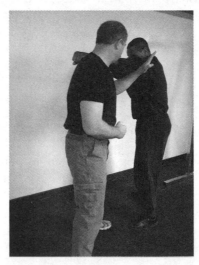

Fig. 4-001: A block is not telegraphed.

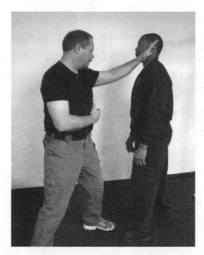

Fig. 4-002: A strike usually is telegraphed, even if it is the exact same motion as the block.

doing to your body. The single critical piece of information is that you are under attack and you must act *now*.

Counter-ambush training bypasses the two middle steps of the OODA loop. It cuts it down to Observe/Act. The system used to train this is Operant Conditioning (OC).

Operant Conditioning is simple. A stimulus is paired with a response. The response you want is rewarded (a smile, "good job, do it again" or just the satisfying thud of well-placed impact). Incorrect responses are punished.* Do not wait for perfection to reward. Reward any improvement so that the trainee develops some momentum towards the goal.

Then train for repetition until the student receives the stimulus and responds immediately without thinking. OC can train a simple response to near reflex speed, sort of an artificial reflex. It does this by cutting out the middle two steps of the OODA loop. There is no Orient, no Decide. You body has trained: X happens, do Y.

---

* Punishment and reward have very specific meaning in Behaviorist psychology. A reward is anything that encourages a specific behavior. A punishment is anything that discourages a behavior. A frown, starting over, or simply not rewarding an effort make it less likely for the effort to be repeated in the same way and so count as punishment. It does not mean beatings or extra push-ups.

Choose the stimulus carefully. Martial arts generally use OC to train, but they train to very specific stimuli. A right hammer fist coming straight down gets a left upper block. Repeat a thousand times and it becomes artificial reflex. Then the left hammer fist matches to the right upper block. Thousands of repetitions. Then the outside block to the straight punch. Thousands more. Training in this way for years can get a student to handle a decent percentage of attacks at something approaching reflex speed.

It does work and many martial artists have a story about responding instantly to a sudden attack. This approach also takes time.

By batching stimuli you can speed the process from years to days or hours. It needs to be reinforced and retrained periodically, but the ability to make a single technique work against many attacks is critical in that first quarter-second. Batching stimuli is simply training that all like attacks can be treated the same. Martial arts that emphasize angles of attack instead of types of attack are a huge step in the right direction.

There are three batch stimuli that I think are critical and two more that are important.

1) *An attack from the front.* Essentially, this is any attack that you see coming or when you can see the Threat after you feel the attack. (You don't always see the attack before you are injured, that's life in the big city.) If the technique is good, whether the attack is right- or left-handed, armed or unarmed, kick or punch should make no difference whatsoever.

2) *A strike or pull off-balance from behind.* I can combine those because what I teach for this works the same on both, as well as weapon retention.

3) *Being overborne from behind.* I don't have a single technique that works both for being yanked from your feet backwards and for being lifted off your feet and rushed forward. If I ever come up with one, this teaching process will get even simpler.

4) *Upward vector.* Less critical perhaps, but I also have something for an upward vector coming at my body, because in my experience that is usually a knife. What I use for option one, above, will work,

but I will likely be stabbed. Don't get hung up on that. Damage is the natural environment of a fight.

If you think for a second that anything in this book or any book intends to get you out of a criminal assault unscathed, put the book down right now and give it some good thinking time. Criminals hurt people to make a living. To get drugs. They take what they want and they are experienced in making that work. An experienced bad guy will always have the edge over an inexperienced good guy. All my book can provide is a few percentage points of advantage and, hopefully, a minimum of bullshit to clog your brain.

5) *Move first.* A fifth technique for closing the distance and neutralizing the Threat when I have the opportunity is to move first. This isn't Operant Conditioning, but just a reminder not to take the pre-emptive move off the table.

Those are the stimuli I suggest that you train for. If you have a specific fear or are aware that your local criminals use a different pattern, design a response for that. Also, drop me a line and let me know what exactly your local bad guys do.

4.1.2: the perfect move

You then have to practice a response to each of these stimuli batches. It must be simple, fast and flexible enough to deal with everything that comes with the stimulus. In my opinion, they should be perfect moves. A perfect move does four things in a single action:

1) It betters your position;
2) It worsens the Threat's position;
3) It protects you from damage; and
4) It damages the Threat or unbalances the Threat if damage isn't justified, but this is counter-assault. If you are ambushed, only enough damage to get out safely is justified.

A move is perfect if it does all four things. It's pretty damn good if it does three. Running away does all of these except to damage the Threat. From a legal standpoint, that is better than perfect. Tactically it is only good if the Threat doesn't chase faster than you run.

To (1) "better your position" is to put you in a place where you can better apply power to the Threat's body.* That means close enough to reach what you need to reach with good enough footing that you can apply power to strike, push or pull, and ideally where you can take advantage of the bad angle in the Threat's foot work. (See Figs. 4-003 through 4-005.)

To (2) "worsen the Threat's position" is to place him (or yourself) in a place or stance where he can't effectively apply power to your body. Creating distance works for this. Snapping his head back or disrupting his balance makes it impossible for him to strike with force until he recovers. Getting behind him or to the flank behind the elbow puts you in a dead zone where it is very difficult for him to attack. (See Figs. 4-006 through 4-008.)

Blocking is essentially reactive and, especially from surprise, it is too slow and takes too much brain to be effective. In order to act to (3) "protect yourself from damage," and nothing is perfectly safe

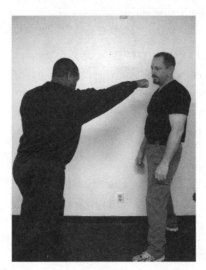

Fig. 4-003: Out of range.

* This is goal-dependent. In the quarter-second of counter-assault you cannot get away. You weren't expecting to be hit so you weren't prepared with a plan for where and how to run. If this were not the case then bettering your position would likely include getting some distance or finding cover.

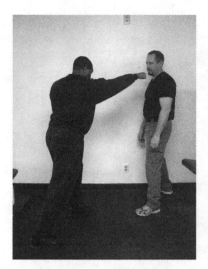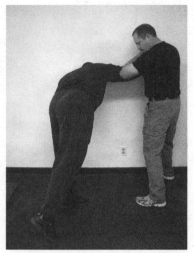

Fig. 4-004A or Fig 4-004B: When you are out of range, reaching just makes your blow ineffective and puts you off balance.

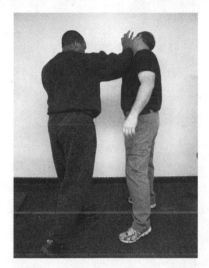

Fig. 4-005: This is good range.

when someone is trying to harm or kill you—the move itself must have defense built into it, safety derived from position and movement.

To (4) "damage the Threat" seems obvious, but with a technique that does not depend on how the Threat is moving or specifically

101

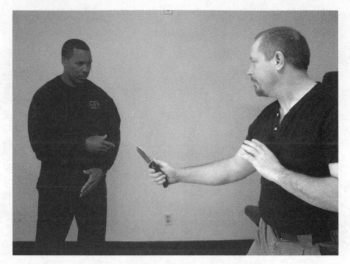

Fig. 4-006: Out of range is safe.

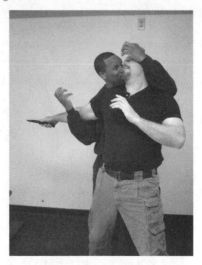

Fig. 4-007: On the flank or behind is safe.

where he is, it takes some applied principles to reliably make an un-aimed and possibly unbalanced attack injure.

Remember also that you must be able to follow it up. It might end the encounter. You have to be ready if it doesn't. Part of bettering your position is leaving yourself in a range of distance where you are an effective fighter.

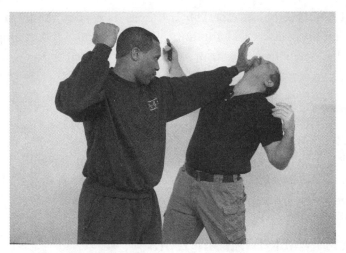

Fig. 4-008: Spine bent isn't bad either.

Keeping this in mind, you will have to design your own responses. I'll describe some of mine here and methods I teach—but not for you to imitate unquestioningly. This is *your* life. *Your safety is your responsibility*. Take permission to create whatever works for you.

The counter-assault techniques will not always end the fight. They will sometimes. Right after I taught the Dracula's Cape for the first time (I was still working on it) an enforcement deputy contacted me, "Dude! The day after you showed that, a guy jumped me and I did the Dracula thingy. Knocked him out!"

That's cool, but the best you can count on is that, properly executed, a counter-assault technique can level the playing field.

When a Threat attacks you, he has a plan and he is counting on your surprise. He is expecting you to freeze in fear and leave him free to do whatever dastardly things he has planned. He expects your own adrenaline to ensure that he wins.

An operant conditioned response will kick in before the adrenaline surge that might trigger freeze rather than fight or flight. Operant Conditioning works at the speed of nerve, hormones at the speed of blood. So it will give you one technique with all your trained speed, power, and precision before the Survival Stress Response kicks in and ruins your fine and complex motor skills.

The OC response, especially if it does damage to the threat, will mess up his plans. It will also force him to reset his OODA loop and start the adrenaline cascade in him that he expected to freeze you. It doesn't ensure that you won't freeze as well, but both of you getting a hormone flood evens the playing field considerably.

4.2: examples

What follows are some examples of OC counter-assault. If some of them resonate with you, that's fine. Don't just mimic though. Figure out why they work and adapt them to be your own.

4.2.1: attack from the front

The simplest counter-assault is palm-heel to the face. There is no defensive move, no block combined with it. Your radar is up, you think something is wrong and suddenly anything comes at you and you give a hard, fast (above all *fast*) palm-heel to the face.

If a weapon or kick is involved you will have to step in with it. I prefer a drop-step, which is essentially a controlled fall. If your strike is properly structured it will transmit the power of your entire falling body weight to the heel of your palm. Most people fall significantly harder than they can punch.

This isn't my personal preferred technique but it is effective for strikers. Does it better your position? Slightly. If you are a striker the palm-heel prevents your attacker from entering too deeply and the drop-step puts you in range to deliver more strikes.

Does it worsen his position? Absolutely. The thing about getting your head snapped back is that it puts the spine in an awkward position where you can't really do anything, at least for an instant.

Palm-heel-to-the-face clearly does damage. Delivered with structure, a drop-step and the proper angle: it can really mess up the cervical spine.

Does it protect you? Yes, and this is an important point:

Amateurs fight bodies. They study bodies, they break down bodies and they train to counter technique. Professionals fight minds. This will come up again later and really the entire section on de-escalation was all about fighting minds—and you are fighting a mind.

Almost everyone chokes when something comes at his or her face. They abort the attack to protect themselves. People will abort a perfectly good punch, baseball bat swing or knife thrust to dodge a paper cup thrown in their face. That defensive flinch is very reliable but it is hard for many people to rely on a purely offensive technique. They want to buy insurance, to put some effort into defense. Just in case.

In the first quarter-second a fast committed single-move offense is better protection than trying to divide your mental and physical resources between offense and defense. I have seen offense consistently protect better than defense in this situation, but I can use nothing but my experience to convince you. Trust your own common sense.

There are two counter-assault techniques that I teach and use for attacks from the front, basically for anything I see coming. One I use naturally when jumped and I have used the other occasionally. I like them. They put me in a good position for very close-range fighting which is my preference, and give me numerous low-damage options which my bosses prefer.

Why two? Damn good question. Thanks for asking. Because there are two common flinch responses for something suddenly flying at your face. Some people duck, turn away, and throw their arm up so that the elbow is roughly between their own face and the Threat. Others, including me, tend to throw both hands up in front of the face palms out. If the technique you train is based on your natural flinch it will be easier to learn.

Both entries use similar footwork. Assume an interview stance (weight evenly balanced, one foot leading so that you have a definite lead side, hands unobtrusively high, perhaps scratching your ear) and turn the lead foot so the toe points slightly inward which protects the groin with minimal movement.

From that stance use the drop-step with whichever foot is closest to the threat. A drop-step starts by suddenly lifting the leg closest to the Threat and falling while launching with the back leg, then catching your self with the lead foot. Using gravity is faster than stepping or lunging. It requires little power and once practiced to proficiency goes un-telegraphed. By maximizing the use of gravity and body mass, even small people can hit hard.

If the drop-step is used to the front or sides, the rear foot slides up to establish a good fighting stance. If you perform the drop-step to the rear, the same thing happens but is accompanied by a turn so that you are facing the Threat.

In the Dracula's Cape response, at the first visual cue or telegraph of an attack, you counter-attack by burying your face in the crook of your lead elbow and drop-stepping into the threat. Tuck your chin and brace your lead hand on your own opposite shoulder which leaves only a thin slit over the eyes vulnerable. You can wrap your off hand around your body to give added protection to your ribs. Properly executed, your entire body weight and leg strength focuses on the point of the elbow which will blow through the Threat's guard or attack and impact, usually on the face if the Threat is short, the sternum if the Threat is tall, or the throat if the Threat is about the same size. On impact, the lead arm can uncoil to control the Threat's neck or slide to slap the ear, while the opposite hand can strike or come up under the Threat's arm to the elbow leverage point and raise the elbow and turn the Threat. You can combine knee strikes with any of these actions. (See Figs. 4-009 through 4-013.)

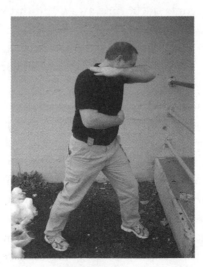

Fig. 4-009: Structure of Dracula's Cape from the side.

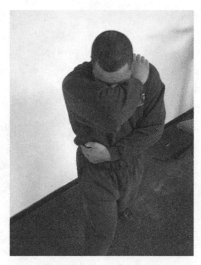

Fig. 4-010: Structure of Dracula's Cape from the front.

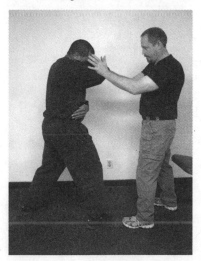

Fig. 4-011: Testing Structure.

The elbow motion in Dracula's Cape is not a swing or a blow, think of it as a thrust. You are jousting. The elbow point leads with a bones-forward armored rush.

Practicing Dracula's Cape safely requires armor and a kicking shield. A few students with both body mass and good technique can blow through that but the gear will provide sufficient protection in

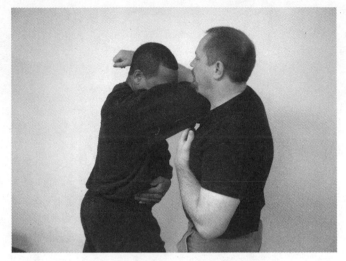

Fig. 4-012: Dracula's Cape in use.

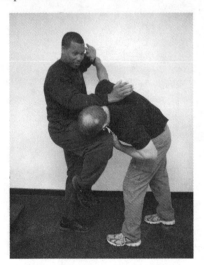

Fig. 4-013: Possible follow-up.

most cases. The student begins by practicing the technique in the air, paying special attention to the structure of the elbow and the drop-step. There should be no preparatory rise before the drop-step; it is a pure falling action.

Once that is acceptable, the student pairs with an armored partner with a kicking shield over the partner's armored chest. (See Fig. 4-014.)

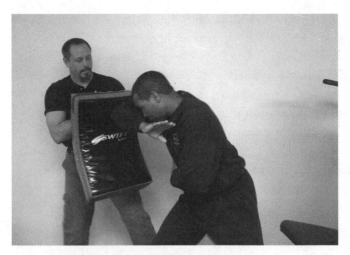

Fig. 4-014: Dracula's Cape practice on kicking shield.

The student will stand at ease or in an interview stance (on-alert but looking relaxed). The partner will then launch an attack-punch, kick or charge (soft weapons are fine if they can hold the shield equally well). The student immediately launches the counter-assault. The force can be considerable. Great care must be taken that the attack cues are realistic and given with intent. You want the student to develop a reflex to defend from an attack, not to cream someone who waves.

The attacks should not be sparring attacks with feints or have any moves to trick the student. A full-blown assault is an onslaught. Feints have no place in it.

Then the student faces three partners spread evenly across his visual field—left flank, center, and right flank. The partners all have armor and kicking shields. One, and only one, will initiate an attack. The student will key on that motion and launch the counter-attack at that Threat immediately. This drill begins training the response to the artificial reflex level.

There is an important training artifact you need to be aware of here. By only practicing the technique, you can inadvertently train the student to stop, to freeze, after the initial counter-assault move.[*]

---

[*] A training artifact is a habit instilled by training that is for the purpose of training, not survival. It is usually a bad habit.

As soon as you are satisfied that the student's technique is good, set the expectation that he or she should continue fighting until it is safe to escape.

The Spearhead Entry is the one that I have found myself using since the first time a boxer tried to take me out. You will see it in many older systems of jujutsu and recognize the bones of it in traditional karate's augmented block. Tony Blauer, a researcher, teacher, innovator (still loving the HighGear armor, Tony) has made a well-researched, modern version the core of his S.P.E.A.R system. See Figs. 4-015 through 4-017.

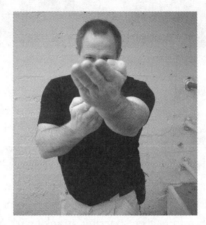

Fig. 4-015: Spearhead structure from front.

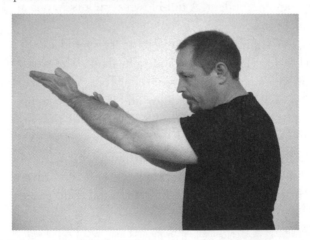

Fig. 4-016: Spearhead structure from side.

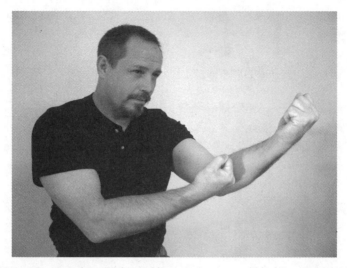

Fig. 4-017: Recognize this? Traditional karate's "augmented block" morote uke. I just use open fingers for gripping.

At the first visual cue or telegraph of an attack, you counter-attack by throwing both hands forward so that the lead hand aims just to the side of the Threat's neck and the back of the rear hand rests with the fingertips on the middle forearm of the lead hand. Both hands are palm-up. Simultaneously, you drop-step, shortening distance on the Threat. The arm position is similar to the bow of an icebreaker and tends to blow through the Threat's guard and/or disrupt any strike he is making. Hips and feet must follow the arms, do not lean into the movement. (See Fig. 4-018.) Properly applied, one of your forearms usually hits the Threat's carotid triangle. The finishing position leaves the Threat vulnerable to neck manipulations and knee strikes to the abdomen, thigh, or knee. (See Fig. 4-019.)

There is more to this than the pictures can illustrate. People who are not infighters tend to leave their hips too far away in both moves, which weaken the technique, compromise balance and make follow-up techniques less effective. With the Spearhead, strong people tend to hit at the collarbone and then push the Threat away sacrificing the range advantage of an infighter.

These pose a lot of potential damage to the Threat. Dracula's Cape focuses a huge amount of power on a tiny point of bone. The Spear

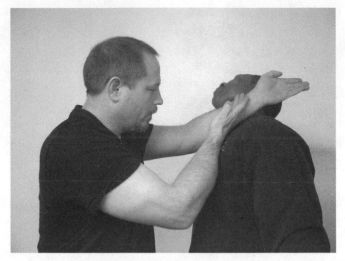

Fig. 4-018: Spearhead entry in use.

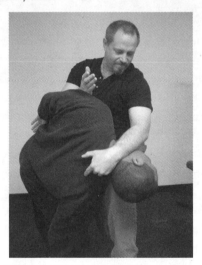

Fig. 4-019: Possible follow-up.

hits the carotid triangle, one of the better stun points in the body. Both give you the spine for the follow-up which infighters love.

This isn't meant to be a picture book or a technique book in any case. Examine Figs. 4-020 through 4-034. Look at what they do and why they work. Because of the combination of a structured shield and closing the distance, they work against a wide variety of technique. The structured shields of the hand position deflect force coming straight at you. Closing the distance neutralizes circular attacks and chokes kicks. Specific kicks are effective only in specific ranges.

Training for Spearhead follows the same protocol as Dracula's Cape except rather than armor, the partner can put his elbows and forearms together, fists up and braced against his or her forehead. This can act as a simulated neck. (See Fig. 4-025.) If you don't practice arm toughening exercises, you may want to invest in some forearm guards.

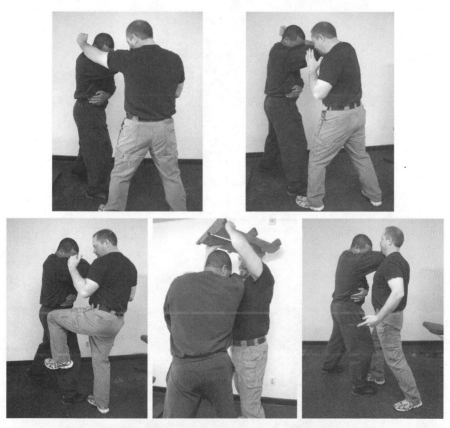

Figs. 4-020 through 4-024: Any counter-assault must work against most things without modification. The same technique spikes right- and left-handed techniques equally. The closing chokes kicks and protects from clubs, bar stools and lumber. There is no guarantee that a knife thrust won't get in, but the damage may make the Threat abort and hopefully will limit the attack to one thrust, instead of eight.

They will take a beating. It may also be necessary for the instructor to stand behind the partner and launch arm attacks to cue the student. (See Fig. 4-026.)

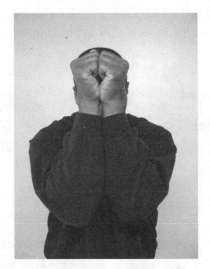

Fig. 4-025: Making an artificial neck for Spearhead practice.

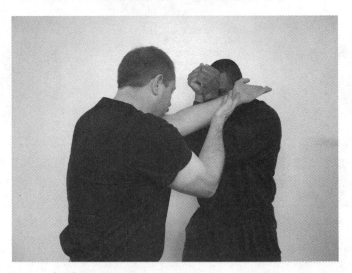

Fig. 4-026: Spearhead practice.

114

4.2.2: attacked from the rear

One of the most common attacks, particularly on women, is to grab from behind by the face or the hair and yank off-balance backwards. They might be yanked upward or thrown down to the ground.

You need to respond quickly and decisively to any unexpected aggressive touch from behind.* The response should be the same whether the attack is a grab, a strike, being yanked off-balance, or even a Threat trying to take your weapon if you are armed. As soon as you feel an unexpected, aggressive touch, you turn toward the point of contact leading with the nearest elbow and drop-step. Use your falling weight on the point of your elbow to deliver the counter-attack. (See Figs. 4-027 through 4-029.) Immediately follow up with strikes, takedowns and spine manipulations, as appropriate, until it is safe to assess the situation.

You turn towards the point of contact because that is your one decisive clue about where the Threat is. The elbow lead can do a lot of damage, a la Dracula's Cape, but sometimes it winds up wrapping the Threat's arms. Doesn't matter, and here is another of the differences between amateurs and professionals in a fight. Amateurs try to make things perfect. Professionals just try to make things better. There are no do-overs so if I wrap the arms or miss entirely, fine. I work from

---

Dracula's Cape and the Spearhead are *irimi*, which is Japanese for entries. Obvious, since the point is to safely close the distance. I'd been cautioned against using Japanese terms when teaching officers, so I just called them entries. That was cool. However, when you are teaching defenses against attacks from behind never tell a room full of cops that you are about to teach them "rear entries." You'll lose a half-hour of class time with the laughing. Hence, the clumsier "counter-assault" phrase.

---

* This is the key stimuli, unexpected aggressive touch. Not a buddy tapping your shoulder or a toddler trying to hold your hand. You know the difference. It is crucial that the stimuli you train with mimic real attacks, that the touches (strikes, grabs) are aggressive.

there, And if I happen to catch the guy just right and he goes down, that's cool too.

Because this already relies on using dropping bodyweight, it is a very small shift to start using being yanked off-balance as an advantage. This will come up again in Chapter 6: The Fight. Combat is a matter of forces and chaos. A poor fighter tries to ignore the forces and the chaos. A good fighter tries to minimize the effects of force vectors and chaos, to fight his own plan. A superior fighter uses the things he can't control to increase his own effective speed and power. Is getting yanked off-balance a negative if you can use the fall to hit with four times your normal power? (See Figs. 4-030 through 4-033.)

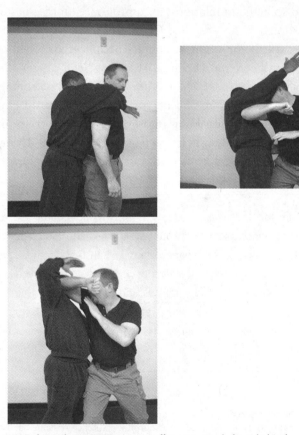

Figs. 4-027 through 4-029: Drop-step elbow to attack from behind.

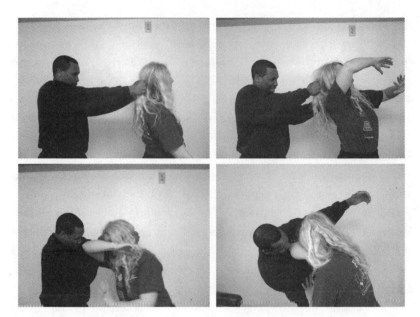

Fig.s. 4-030 through 4-033: One of the few techniques that works when the victim is grabbed by the hair from behind and lifted off her feet. She utilizes her own falling weight.

A key safety point to training this technique is keeping one hand up to protect the jaw and ear on the side that you grab your partner.

This technique will give you a chance to recover from a strike from behind, a stranglehold (if you act on contact, not waiting for

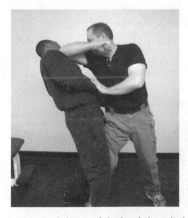

Fig. 4-034: With the retention capabilities of the level three holster we have found it more effective and safer to concentrate on neutralizing the Threat while he has a hand tied-up rather than wrestling for the weapon.

the Threat to get a good grip), weapon grabs and even stabs (the first stab will get in before you notice, remember your goal is to prevent the next eight). However, it is ineffective if the Threat grabs you and rushes you off your feet forward, like a bum's rush or bear-hugs you and rams you into a wall.

The defense I prefer in those cases is very simple, but very difficult to practice safely. If you feel yourself lifted off your feet *forward*, you latch on to whatever is gripping you and go limp.

Suddenly going limp takes a little practice, but even very strong people have trouble lifting a giant rag doll. Suddenly going limp makes you drop, usually in front of the Threat's moving knees. He will fall. If you have latched onto his arms, the Threat will be unable to control the fall. A face-plant or landing on the point of the shoulder is likely. I still remember the young man who was thrown with his arms trapped. Despite the soft mats, his clavicle was shattered.

The counter-assault stage is a quarter of a second of any fight. In one way or another, you have been working on your ethical issues since birth. Civilization has been working on legalities since the advent of writing. Criminals have been polishing their skills since they were old enough to take other kids' milk money. Your ability to avoid, escape, or defuse may take seconds or spread over hours.

The actual assault, when it happens, will begin in an instant and it will be over in a fraction of a second. What you do here will determine how you are positioned for the next two stages. Whatever you do, it has to be effective and it has to be fast.

CHAPTER 5: THE FREEZE

Ralph was a veteran fighter, both skillful and experienced. Also a pretty nice guy with good awarenes and good verbal skills. As a sergeant he had excellent rapport with both inmates and other officers. He was just doing his job.

An inmate took his words, his expression, something as an insult. This was an inmate who had honed the blitz attack to a fine art. Ralph was hit three times before he was aware an assault was underway. Then his first instinct was to grab the Threat to try to slow down the situation and buy time to think.

It all ended well. There was a fair amount of blood, mostly from the Threat. Ralph's injuries were cosmetic. The other 56 or 57 inmates watching chose not to get involved. Minor injuries all around.

The sergeant was mentally torturing himself for a long time. Because he froze. It wasn't much of a freeze—three hits for an average blitz attack is less than half a second. He'd turn it over in his mind, wondering how he let his guard down and how the Threat had opportunity and why he didn't see or feel it happening in time to react.

This is the thing, the difference between a fight and an assault, the victim is behind the curve, trying to play catch up, trying to figure out what the situation is and how to respond while the Threat is already well into the steps of his plan. This is where you start in an assault: fifteen points behind, halfway into the fourth quarter, and you don't know if you're playing basketball or football and you aren't dressed for either game.

Because he's done this for decades, Ralph thought he should have done better. He's alive and mostly uninjured. The Threat was dragged away in cuffs. It honestly doesn't end much better than that. But that freeze, that half-second, didn't let him rest for a long time.

If you play with snakes long enough, you get bit. It's natural. But the human animal has to ask "why me, why that time, why, why, why?" A skilled officer will prevent 99% of what could happen, but when that 1% breaks through, he can feel like a rookie all over again.

Ralph did well. We all hate it, but freezing is normal and natural, and bad guys rely on it, they expect it to last for the entire assault. Anyone who thinks they can't be surprised or won't freeze for an instant when they are caught off-guard is wrong.

Whether you did well in the counter-assault phase or not, the next thing you will do is freeze. If you are lucky or well-trained, the Operant Conditioning may have kicked-in and the Threat may be down, lying on the ground trying to figure out what just happened. If things *didn't* go so well, you may be the one lying on the ground as boots slam into your ribs, wondering what just happened and trying to remember what to do next and suddenly concerned with remembering your first girlfriend's eye color . . . *what a horrible thing to die forgetting*, your mind whispers.

I can almost guarantee that you will freeze. Whether it lasts a fraction of a second or for the short remainder of your time on earth will depend on a combination of your nature, your training, and your experience.

5.1: biological background

Behavioral biology lists three survival responses to sudden extreme stress, the "three Fs": Fight, Flight, and Freeze. Dave Grossman lists four: Fight, Flight, Posture, and Submit.[*] All *five* of the listed responses, Fight, Flight, Freeze, Posture, and Submit are hard-wired reactions to an immediate, serious, living threat.[**]

The hard-wired fight response is nothing like a Monkey Dance or sparring fight and nothing like the way a predator attacks. In this

---

[*] Grossman, Dave.

[**] The responses to major disasters are quite different, more limited and predictable. See *The Unthinkable* by Amanda *Ripley*.

context, "fight" is the thrashing of prey when all hope is pretty much lost. It is not systematic or skilled, but a flailing of hooves or gnashing teeth that might bite or might just grab air. If your Survival Stress Response, your cocktail of fear hormones, kicks up high enough, this is the kind of fighting your body and hindbrain will be driving you to, no matter how hard or realistically you have trained.

The hard-wired flight response is a blind panic run. People do stumble and fall like in horror movies because the SSR destroys their coordination. They are too blinded by tunnel-vision to see their own feet as they run and they are so focused on the danger, which is behind them, that frequently the victim will run full-force into an electrical pole, a tree, or into traffic.

This chapter is all about freezing and breaking out of the freeze. There are many reasons to freeze and many different flavors of freezing. The hard-wired response is a survival mechanism based in the simple fact that predators notice movement. If you don't move, you might not be seen and therefore you might live.

Posturing and submitting are the two bases of the Monkey Dance and to some extent, all social violence. Humans usually don't want to hurt other humans. It's inefficient and dangerous. Whether the human seeks respect or fear or status or money, it is much easier and safer to scare someone into submission than to beat them into submission.

Posture is sending the aggressive signals: the hard stare, the verbal challenge . . . all the way up to the shock and awe of an artillery bombardment. Remember that you are fighting minds not bodies. Artillery bombardment or fistfight, you rarely destroy 100% of the Threat's capability to fight. Instead, you destroy his will.

Individuals, unless you shut down their brainstem or break every long bone in their body, can still fight. Nations and organizations can keep fighting unless you kill everyone old enough to pull a trigger. In any case, individuals or nations are rarely beaten. They give up.

Posturing, making yourself look intimidating, influences the enemy to give up. A good posture influences the other to submit, and that is the best bet. Contrast that to *this* reaction to violence: "Don't hurt me, don't hurt me, I'll do anything you say just please don't hurt me." There is a body language that goes with it, a dropping of eye contact, a shrinking into oneself. You will see it in a beaten child and you will see it in the eyes of a starving man who has given up.

It should be clear right away that there are two different mechanisms in play and that they evolved for different situations. The three Fs are hard-wired reactions to predators. Not predators in the sense of criminals, but looking up and seeing a bear much too close, most people freeze. Freezing is the most common response because it is the safest. A few run, which sometimes works but often triggers the chase instinct in a predator. I have never seen or heard of anyone whose first instinct was to fight when surprised by a large carnivore. That response seems to be a last resort only when you are out of places to run and the teeth close on you.

These responses work in their intended environment when humans are attacked by a different species. The things that make you clumsy when you are terrified—sensory distortion, blood drawn from the limbs to the center body—are advantages when you are being eaten. The blood drawn to the core means the predator can chew on your arms and legs and you won't bleed out quickly. Sensory distortion, with everything feeling and sounding far away and muted is a godsend if the feelings and sounds are teeth tearing your flesh and crushing your bones. Remember that, typically, animals are alive during the early stages of being eaten.

Even the high-end ultimate terror response, going catatonic and voiding your bladder and bowels, is a survival strategy. A predator knows what dead is. People have survived bear attacks by playing dead. For example in 2008, Brent Case was mauled by a 900-pound grizzly in British Columbia. Mr. Case credits playing dead for his survival. A bear has intelligence and will sometimes save food for later, when it might be softer.

A mouse that is still scurrying, even weakly, is entertaining for a cat. The one that has given up and only wants to die will sometimes live, because the cat gets bored with the mouse and distracted by something else.

Do not interpret what I am saying as being high-percentage strategies. They aren't . . . but when circumstances are really, really bad, low-percentage strategies are better than nothing. And, there are NO high-percentage strategies to survive being eaten. They are hard-wired because over a billion years of evolution even partial percentage points are worth the advantage.

Posture and Submit are hard-wired for social interactions. The Monkey Dance, of course, and all of that . . . but even war. The Napoleonic column was an inefficient way to use musketmen. The math didn't work as only the relatively small front could fire and they couldn't reload. A line across their path, also armed with muskets, could put much more fire on the column . . . but the columns were effective for a very long time because they were visually intimidating. The mathematically superior lines tended to break and run in fear.

If killing won wars we'd still be using bows. A good soldier with a muzzleloader could fire three times a minute. I am a mediocre archer and I can fire twelve arrows a minute easily. Up until the early or mid-1800s, the bow was more accurate and had a much greater range than the firearms available. But they didn't make smoke and fire and thunder. They didn't scare men and terrify horses . . . and wars are never won by killing people, they are won by breaking will.

This posture/submit cycle is universal across social violence.

The other thing to distinguish is that you can consciously mimic any of the hard-wired responses and use them *as a strategy*.

Trying to establish social dominance is a remarkably poor idea beyond your species, especially heading up the food chain. Submit to a shark and you will probably be eaten. But many people have tried to make themselves look big and loud and succeeded in convincing a predator to go away using posturing cross-species. Playing dead or even faking a heart attack or a seizure has stopped or circumvented incidents of violence, including the Group Monkey Dance. I can't count the number of times I have befriended a "dangerous" dog by showing puppy/playful body language.

5.2: what freezing is

Freezing is the state of not moving when you are in danger. Sometimes it is involuntary as your adrenaline kicks in and you go into hard-wired freeze mode. Sometimes it is a strategy: you choose not-moving because it is your best option. Sometimes, in the midst of a freeze you honestly can't tell if you can't move or just don't want to.

Perception under extreme stress is altered, both your senses and your awareness of time. I have a report at home from a cell entry on a barricaded, armed threat. From the time the door was opened until I shot, I remember about 3 seconds of stuff. The team leader remembers about a minute of stuff including a conversation that never happened. The rest of the stack wrote it as almost instantaneous.

The team leader was more adrenalized than I was. He perceived a very quick event to take a lot of time and his brain nicely made up some stuff to fill in the details. (Your brain will do this to you. Don't be surprised. It is one of the primary reasons that you should not talk to anyone official immediately after a critical incident.)

I was pretty adrenalized, but I was in the zone. Did it take three seconds? It would take me three seconds right now to do what I did there: scan, aim, reject target, acquire another target, aim, fire, rack a round, then, step out of the way . . . but in the zone? The rest of the team was probably right. It was quick.

The point is that some of the people who see themselves in slow motion or even frozen were in fact moving, or were frozen for only a fraction of what they remember as a long time. And some people who clearly remember doing lots of stuff actually stood frozen with red-hot imaginations. Personal reports of events, particularly freezes, are very unreliable.

5.3: types of freezes

There are many reasons to freeze, many ways to freeze and each type has different implications. Some are relatively easy to train away, some can only be minimized, some disappear entirely. Some freezes feel like freezes. Some don't. And some don't even register with you consciously. You must understand the problem before you can understand the solution, and freezing—a big problem—is not well-understood in humans.

5.3.1: tactical freezes

Tactical Freezing is a *choice*. You freeze on purpose to either: go unnoticed, let the Threat calm down, or to gather information.

Sometimes it is a very good idea not to move. Predators key on motion. Not-moving allows them to move on to something else. This is the basis of the hard-wired freeze response. When you *decide* to do this, *hoping not to be noticed*, it is a tactical freeze. However, you must recognize when you *are* noticed and respond appropriately.

There is a dynamic in survival situations where the old primitive part of your brain says, "Still alive, don't change anything." Even when your conscious brain recognizes circumstances have changed, the hindbrain will try to keep you from changing anything. The first battle to move may be with your self.

Freezing is also a good tactical decision when you are making matters worse. As an old friend used to say, "When a wise man figures out he's in a hole, he stops digging." In a social violence situation a tactical freeze may allow the Threat to *cool down*. It is not a good strategy after damage starts. It is also not something that works if you continue to antagonize or challenge with your body language.

The third possible purpose of a tactical freeze is *information gathering*. If your intuition tingles it may be a good time to stop, look, listen, and smell. Then evaluate and plan.

5.3.2: physiological freezes

I think I can identify two distinct kinds. *When the body switches from its normal metabolic state to an adrenalized state, there's a little tremor as described by Marc MacYoung in "The Professional's Guide to Ending Violence Quickly".* It is literally a new mind and body and there is a slight freeze while you switch gears.

Just as the engine is not powering the wheels between gears, you will not be doing anything while you switch from your oblivious nine-to-five mind into survival mode. Some people switch gears faster than others. The last stage of training with counter-assault is to continue from technique to immediately transition to fight mode. That is how you train to make the gear switch freeze as brief as possible.

Another tactic works when you have recognized a risk. You create a viable plan and a "go button." "If this kicks off (go button) I am sprinting for that door (plan)." It presets your body and mind to switch gears.

The second is when the danger is so overwhelming, or appears to be, that it triggers *the hard-wired freeze response* of "I couldn't move." Sometimes with the loss of bladder control and everything else. This is the deer in the headlights or the baby bird so terrified it sits in your hands in a near-coma. There are many levels of this.

Know that the hard-wired freeze response is triggered by fear, but it doesn't usually feel that unpleasant, kind of warm and floaty with a sound in your ears like the ocean. People who have been so terrified they couldn't move have described this state and decided that they weren't really afraid so they weren't really frozen. It just seemed like a good idea at the time not to move.

Unless you are familiar with this sensation you may be completely frozen and not know it.

5.3.3: non-cognitive mental freeze

The mental freezes are when decisions or thought patterns, or interruptions in thought patterns, keep you from acting. Non-cognitive freezes are deeper than the cognitive, rooted in problems with habits rather than with decisions or thinking. Lots of freezes are mental, which doesn't mean that they are all cognitive.

Lonnie Athens[*] posits that one of the reasons that change is hard is that no matter how screwed-up your life, how horribly you are being victimized or how clear it is that death is inevitable on your current path, you are alive. Your subconscious mind, especially if it has seen a lot of death, is very well aware that your big plan to change your life is only that, a plan. Subconsciously it knows that planning is a game, *this* is real and it will try to stick to what works. Lonnie Athens called this problem *working from the blueprint*. Any time that you attempt

---

[*] *Athens.*

to deal with a dangerous situation from a training perspective for the first time, you will get this freeze.

If your Operant Conditioning response was good, you may have bought the time to get over it, but now you have to deal with the fact that your hindbrain was indulging the child by letting you take all those martial arts classes and didn't believe any of it. You will have to consciously force yourself to act. In my experience, on the second successful action the hindbrain will relent and you can act.

Interestingly, this freeze is easy to corroborate from another area of critical operations, Emergency Medical Technicians and combat medics, and they have a mechanism for beating it. At the end of 91A school at Fort Sam Houston, I could get to a simulated helicopter crash and supervise or conduct the triage, treatment, and evacuation of eight casualties under fire without breaking a sweat. Months later, I was talking to a young lady who suddenly had a seizure and fell hitting her head on the stairs. I froze for a second like a babbling idiot. Often, you will hear similar stories from medics describing the first "real one."

The trick they use to beat the freeze is to talk themselves through it: "What am I supposed to be doing? Ah, err, RABC! Yeah, that's it! Are you okay? Check the airway . . ." Just a couple of moves into what they have trained to do, they get into the zone. The first few seconds are sloppy, then after that, they can use their skills. I found the same thing true in my first fights.

A related phenomenon is *behavioral looping*, doing the same thing endlessly when it is clear that it is not working. Sometimes tragically, even when it is very clear to an objective outsider that the action will certainly lead to death.* The mechanism is the same—death may be in the air, but the hindbrain only knows that what you are doing has not gotten you killed *and any change might*.

---

* Georgia Deputy Kyle Dinkheller was killed January 12, 1988. Even as the killer, who described himself as a Vietnam combat veteran was loading a rifle, Deputy Dinkheller kept repeating verbal commands. Though it was clear (watching the video) where this was going, he didn't shoot the killer when he needed to.

Switching maps is the slight hesitation freeze it takes to adjust to a change in situation. When you think you know what you are dealing with, (e.g., handcuffing a resistive but not dangerous drunk) and it suddenly becomes apparent that you were wrong (a knife gouges your stomach) it takes a small amount of time to switch modes. Changing gears again.

5.3.4: cognitive freezes

Cognitive Freezes are the thought process errors that can make you freeze.

If too much information is coming in, like a flurry of blows, you can be caught in the *Observation Orientation bounce* (From Col. John Boyd's OODA loop) getting new Observations before you have Oriented to the ones you already have prevents you from ever Deciding or Acting. You get stuck continuously trying to Orient to new Observations, and in an assault, each of those Observations is likely to mean damage to you.

The training strategy for this is to use the OO bounce as a stimulus in Operant Conditioning. The batch stimulus becomes getting overwhelmed, the response is either leave the area or shut down the source. Remember that you cannot effectively OC train two responses to one stimulus, so choose wisely.

Novelty. If you can't figure out what is happening, you can't formulate a response to it. So, you can't finish the Orient step of the OODA loop. As with any of the cognitive freezes, don't think of this as purely a logic problem. It happens in a cascade of chemical fear. The phenomenon of "my life passed before my eyes" could be the brain's attempt to scan memory for something that relates to the situation you are in.

Two examples of this from my own experience: face contact, especially open-handed, among adults is a very strong taboo in our culture. When it happens it is a sign of great dominance or great intimacy. Criminals use this sometimes opening an attack with a "bitch slap" that reliably makes people freeze and fall into a submissive mindset.

For most people, the last time they were slapped was as a child being punished. The mind falls back to that mindset.

The second example: there is rarely a physiological reason to collapse when shot, barring brainstem or spine compromise, but I have seen officers in training not actually injured at all, collapse and play dead when shot. After all, the only time they have been "shot" before was playing cops-n-robbers as kids and if you don't die, you're a cheater. Are the officers who choose to "die" in training the same officers who collapse and bleed out from non-lethal wounds in real life?

These examples were relatively novel because there had been no new valid information since childhood. Extreme novelty, like using a cat as a weapon, can make for a harder freeze.

Novelty can cross over the line into *cognitive dissonance*. If your expectations of a fight do not match what you see, your brain is almost compelled to sort it out and come to an understanding. If the fight you are in doesn't look, feel, or sound like the fight you have trained for, you will freeze. This, in my opinion, is compounded in martial artists who are very certain that their training has prepared them for reality.

The next two are very closely related. One of the Tactical Freezes is in order to gather intelligence. This is only appropriate before damage happens. Once boots are flying or weapons are in play you need to be doing something. One of the most common reported freezes is the victim trying to figure out *why*. Processing the experience is something you can do later, when you are safe. In the moment of assault, moving is required, not understanding.

Very similar is the desire to come up with a *plan* before acting. Each second spent planning is a second of damage. Damage decreases your ability to execute plans. You can easily die, doing nothing, while groping for the perfect plan.

5.3.5: social cognitive freezes

The Social Cognitive Freezes are what happens when you attempt to apply your internalized set of civilized rules to an uncivilized situation, when what you expect is not what you see. This is the freeze that you get when you find yourself on the other side of the looking glass.

Lack of confidence falls under this heading. If the person believes, on any level, that his training is flawed or unrealistic, that will increase the hindbrain's reluctance to work off the blueprint. This is not always a bad freeze, bad training *can* make situations worse. If the person believes that he or she doesn't have what it takes, that can become a self-fulfilling prophecy.

The obvious solution is to instill confidence. Become a cheerleader. Tell your students they can do anything. That cure is almost as bad as the problem. It is far easier to instill confidence than competence.

Instill *competence*. Train hard. If you play hard with actual moving bodies, actual impact, if you take hard hits and give them, you might still have this doubt before the fight . . . but once the fight is on, hoo-boy. After spending years training with college athletes, I thought the violent criminal in my first real fight felt like he was made of cheese. I've taken a hit to the face and thought, "Hey, my wife hits harder than you!" If the competence is there, trust that the confidence will come.

Mauricio Machuca's observations on capability and *capacity* were mentioned in the first section. Once again, everything connects. Working out your glitches, finding your limitations and either overcoming them or adapting your training to them pays off here when you can avoid a deadly freeze.

As an instructor, you must be aware that it is almost impossible to tell if a capacity has actually changed in a training environment. It is more likely that the person has only convinced him or herself that training is just a game and it's okay to pretend to eye-gouge. If so, the freeze is hiding there waiting to be triggered.

I sometimes use the analogy of "slipping the leash." Some people either do not have the capacity or it takes extraordinary provocation. Capacity can change under certain provocations. I've done it and I've heard of many other instructors who motivated a woman in a self-defense class who was not effectively defending herself by telling her that the bad guy was coming after her children.

The person's identity itself, through the mechanism of *denial*, can also prevent him or her from acting. Whether it is, "I'm not the sort of person this happens to, this isn't happening," or the equally devastating, "I know what I should do, but I'm not the kind of person who would." The identity, the perception the victim has, prevents action. Even, sometimes, at the cost of life.

Your identity is pretty much an illusion anyway, if it was as solid as people like to believe moods wouldn't exist. You have the power in the moment to be anything you want or need to be. Just take the power.

Ambivalence is a situation that Freud would love. It is the word for when what you want and what is expected of you or what you believe yourself to be come into direct conflict. You really want to clobber your brother-in-law but you don't want to listen to your sister bring it up for the next ten years. Less flippant, this is what happens when an officer involved in a deadly force situation starts thinking about lawsuits and the internal affairs process during a life-or-death encounter.

Desmond Morris mentioned alphas pushing betas until the beta fights and that the resultant injury could weaken the alpha to the point that his status was in jeopardy. The resulting equation, fear of injury versus desire to maintain dominance over the beta, would tend to freeze the alpha.

I disagree. In a healthy society the alpha doesn't maintain his position through physical domination. I think the glitch/hesitation equation will come from the fact that going physical with an underling at all shows that the alpha is insecure in his position. Provoking the conflict would compound that. The alpha in that example has a lot to lose, not from the physical injuries making him vulnerable but from his own actions eroding his reputation.

As people grow up in society, they learn a variety of skills to deal with conflict. But that is conflict between civilized people, low-level social violence. When faced with a true predator who does not care about society's rules or who the victim is, it is an entirely different world. I call this the "*looking glass effect.*" The rules—the social rules, how your brain and body work, what you have been taught about how to handle other people, or what people value—no longer apply.

Suddenly finding yourself in an alien culture where you don't know the rules and your life is at stake creates a pretty deep panic

131

reaction. All of the physiological reasons can combine with information gathering and denial to make you a gibbering wreck.

5.3.6: the pure social freeze

Some people are trained to freeze, conditioned to be victims. It probably started as or was intended to be submission but the programming has gone far deeper. This *trained helplessness* is a survival strategy for long-term abuse where the abuser chooses to see any sign of independence or spirit as an affront to his social status. I have seen the effects of this training but there are people far more qualified to write about the process and implications than I am. The similarities between some of the abuse stories and what the victims became have eerie parallels in Elie Wiesel's "Night."

5.4: breaking the freeze

Many of the types mentioned above came with training advice. There are some types of freezes that you can eliminate or minimize in training. The more different things you experience, the fewer novelty freezes you will have. The better you know your glitches, the fewer capacity freezes you will have.

You will still freeze, however. I don't know under what circumstances or how deeply or for how long, but the freeze is there, even in experienced fighters who get ambushed. I have even felt the freeze after the event. When everything was over. I have caught myself standing, staring, trying to remember what I was supposed to do next. Freezes happen.

In order to break the freeze, you must recognize that you are frozen. If you believe or know you should be doing something and you aren't, you are frozen. If you are taking damage or seeing someone else take damage and you have a warm, comfortable feeling and hear a rushing noise in your ears like the ocean, you are frozen.

Recognize it. Acknowledge it. Say, "I'm frozen." Out-loud is better because it reminds you that you can affect the world. It is easy to say stuff in your head and not do it. Then tell yourself to do something—scream, hit back, run—and do it. Then, again, tell yourself to do something, maybe even repeat the same action and do it.

This is the same mechanism as the medic talking himself through his first real trauma call.

This is something that I've back-engineered. It is not theory so much as looking back at the times I was frozen and should have gotten hurt badly and didn't and figuring out how I made myself move.

Step 1. Recognize you are frozen.

Step 2. Make yourself do something.

Step 3. Repeat Step 2.

In my experience and double-checking with my BTDT (Been There, Done That) friends, this method seems universal. Professionals still freeze. This is how they unfreeze. We can't know whether the ones who failed to unfreeze tried this and it didn't work. We can't know for sure if this can be taught, or if just reading it here is enough for you to use it when the time comes. I hope so.

5.5: anti-freeze habit

There is one thing that helps with breaking freezes and real fights in general. It is also a life habit that can profoundly affect what you accomplish in life and how your friends see you. It can make your reputation.

Develop the habit of doing unpleasant things quickly and without hesitation. If you are going to jump in the cold water, jump in the cold water. If you need to get up, get your ass out of bed. Do the dishes that need doing. Finish the hard jobs at work while everyone else is coming up with excuses to get out of them.

Like with applying force, all of your agonizing should be concentrated on deciding *if* you should do something. Once that is decided, do it. Quickly, efficiently, and without hesitation.

The ability to do this amazes mere mortals. It almost qualifies as a super-power.

CHAPTER 6: THE FIGHT

The Threat was walking out of the casino. He seemed to be complying. He didn't like it but he had been ordered to leave and he was leaving.

Suddenly he jumped in the air and spun, swinging a wild punch. I ducked and his fist sailed over my head to connect solidly with my partner's jaw. It made a meaty, slapping noise.

The Threat landed and for one second I had the perfect opening—his ribs were exposed, he was leaning slightly away with a roulette table on the other side to keep him from falling away—and I had a thunderous sidekick. The advantages were the problem. We were there to throw out this guy, not to smash his ribs against a table. I let the moment slip away.

When it was all over, after a wrestling match under the roulette table, I shakily pulled myself to my feet thinking, "Damn. That wasn't anything like sparring."

You worked out your ethical and legal knowledge long ago. You understand criminals and recognize an ambush or a set-up. You couldn't avoid this one, couldn't defuse it. The strike came out of nowhere and you taste blood in your mouth. You might have counter-assaulted. You don't know. You don't remember. For a second you hesitated, not sure what to do, but you broke through that . . .

Once the freeze is broken, the fight is on.

Whatever you have trained in martial arts or defensive tactics now has a chance to work. You have to get here, however. Preferably in one piece.

This could be the longest chapter in the book. By rights, it could run to millions of pages just repeating what everyone else has ever written about fighting and self-defense. But this isn't a technique manual. It is a guidebook to something that is a very strange country for most people. I am going to introduce you to how the rules change once you step through the looking glass.

There are four elements in every fight: you, the threat or threats, the environment, and luck. What you think you know about those four elements may be very different on the other side of the looking glass.

In this section we will cover some of the elements of using force in actual application that are obvious to insiders and may be new to you. Also, you will find some of the concepts presented in the section on Freezing reintroduced in the context of The Fight. It is unrealistic to discuss any fight scenario without discussing freezing.

6.1: you

You have certain expectations about who you are, how you think and what your body can do. If you have trained in martial arts, combat or self-defense, these expectations may run very deep. They have become part of your identity.

Unless you have experienced violence and chaos, these things that you believe are assumptions. They are not facts. Remember the section on Beliefs, Values, Morals, and Ethics? What is coming next might hit you at the belief level. If it does, you may feel it as a personal attack.

When I use "fight" in this section I specifically mean using force to escape from an assault. I do not mean any kind of mutual combat or Monkey Dance stuff. You are under assault. That means that you have been attacked without provoking it. That means that you could not avoid the assault, couldn't run from the assault and couldn't talk your way out of the assault. You are under assault, and the only option you have left is to fight your way out.

Feel free to draw distinctions between fighting and combat and assault survival, *if the distinctions help you clarify your ethics*. But do not get hung up on words. When someone is trying to take your life it isn't about words.

It is not. If your only exposure to violence is in training or books or films, you have only seen pictures of a house. I live in the house.

Give me a chance to show you a few things that all the pictures seem to miss.

6.1.1: this is your brain on fear

You should be aware on some level about how many different people you are and how many different minds you use every day. The mind on a first date is not the same mind as the one that looks at your wife over the breakfast table twenty years later. The mind you are in when you are playing with children or petting a puppy is not the same mindset as keeping an eye on a rival at work.

The way your brain feels when you are doing something that scares you (heights or caves or, for me, swimming in murky water known to have snakes, caimans, and carnivorous fish . . . brrrr) is different than the brain that watches the TV. For that matter, your third or tenth time listening to machine guns fire in the night doesn't even affect your sleep.

You have all of these minds and you have many more you haven't experienced yet. Be thankful for some of that. It is very likely that the mind you will have on the other side of the looking glass will be far different than any of the others. It is hard to use that mind the *first* time and that is unfortunate because the stakes can be very, very high.

We've discussed a lot of what goes on in the chapter on Freezing. Probably the most damaging mental habits you will bring from the normal world are the desire to gather too much information and the perceived need to make a plan.

You need to know that you are taking damage or about to take damage. You need to know what you can do about it—running routes or his available targets and your available weapons. Almost anything beyond that is time wasting.

It is true that with more information you can choose a more efficient plan, but:
- Gathering information takes time
- Time is damage

- You can't often tell in an instant what information will help.

During hostage negotiations, we put people to work finding out all that they can about the Threat to help the primary negotiator build rapport, but we can't tell whether the Threat's love of fishing or his favorite dog or the fact that his mother abused him will be the key in this particular incident. Not all information is useful in a given moment and sometimes you have to gather a lot to find the good stuff. Then you have to identify the good stuff. That all takes time. And, as I said before, time is damage.

In the normal world, most time crunches come from artificial deadlines you miss by a few minutes or hours you might get yelled at. An incoming knife is a very short deadline with far more serious consequences.

How do professionals deal with the time/information problem? They recognize when they have time, gather all the information they can and when it is time to move, they move. Right then. With the information they have.

When a bad guy is interviewing me, trying to work himself up to a Status Seeking Show (usually) or an assault (rarely) . . .* I can almost always talk it down, but every second of listening and talking is matched with watching. Where are his hands? Any weapons? Which side forward? Is a leg loaded? Who is watching? Members of his gang? How many? What is the mood of the crowd? What can he reach me with if he attacks this instant?

If he moves, I move. No matter how much or little time I had to figure out what is going on. Up until that time though, don't waste a second.

The second bad habit is planning. When I am responding, e.g., running to back-up after an officer's assistance call on the radio or paged out with my team, I have some time to plan. Sometimes very little (sprinting to back-up), sometimes a lot. If no one is being injured and there are no hostages I will slow down an operation and, if possible, bore the criminal into surrendering.

---

* Actually, SSS and assaults are very similar in effect and dynamic They need to be differentiated because the motives and thus the de-escalations are different.

Just like fire or earthquake evacuation, it is bad to start planning after the alarm goes off. It is damage to start planning after the fists come in.

Planning in chaos is not all that effective anyway. Bad guys rarely do exactly what is expected and officers die when they stay on a plan after circumstances have changed. Even if you have a plan, even if it is a good one, even if it has worked for you in the past you must be able to walk away and improvise the second the world quits looking like the plan.

Those are merely mental habits. There is more and it is deeper and harder. Your brain chemistry changes under the Survival Stress Response (SSR). Parts of your brain that normally only come out for food and sex want to exert their seniority and run your body the way they used to run it when saber-toothed tigers roamed the savannah and that part of your brain can take over completely.

There are lots of different ways that it can manifest and they seem to vary by who you are and how intense the situation is. Sometimes there is a blur: you remember nothing until it is all over and you look around and you did really, really well. Sometimes you remember details, usually irrelevant details with exquisite sharpness and everything seemed to go in slow motion. You remember everything.

You don't remember it all that accurately though, and you'll see that if you ever get a chance to compare your memory with a video. These aren't sensory distortions, in my opinion, so much as memory distortions. The conscious part of the brain is completely submerged (blur, no memory) or distracted (ultra-sharp focus on worthless detail) so that the more primitive parts of the brain can get things done.

Used to be that every time I got hit in the face, I got the rushing noise and the warm floaty feeling. I had to fight back to the surface to stay in the fight and it felt like swimming up stream. I've gotten used to it so it happens less.

Really, really stupid thoughts pop into your head. In one of the more serious fights I was in (cornered, two on one, no back-up, no one even knew) I suddenly became obsessed with trying to remember what flavor my wedding cake was. My wife liked it better than me worrying about what color my first girlfriend's eyes were, but it was still . . . weird.

Some thoughts are more normal like fear of being sued or concerns about what will happen to your family if you die. These thoughts are still distractions. It's a platitude, but you have to do what you have to do.

The behavioral looping mentioned in "freezes" can also kick in. The old part of your brain that wants to deal with saber-tooths also deals with rhythm and ritual and superstition. You might find yourself doing or saying the same things over and over again when it is clearly not working. You lock into a mental loop.

Rhythm is comforting, as you know if you have ever been so messed up that you wanted to sit in a dark room and rock and hum. That's old brain stuff. It becomes ritual, too, in that even though hitting the big guy in the chest isn't doing anything you've been at it for five seconds and you are still alive. The old part of your brain starts believing that it is a magic charm that keeps death away.

People who get locked in these loops tend to stay in them until they are seriously injured. But that is bad since, of course, injury makes it harder for you to do anything effective.

It takes an act of will to do what you are trained to do. If you have already broken the freeze, you know that you have the will. You must exert your will and keep exerting it until you are safe.

6.1.2: and this is your body

The physiological freeze section covered some of the effects of the Survival Stress Response, specifically that blood is pulled towards the vital organs so that getting a limb chewed is less likely to kill you.

That has some other side effects. You get clumsy is the big one. The strength of your chemical dump will determine how clumsy. Even under a relatively mild dump (and those are rare, unless you have been ambushed a lot and kind of expected this one) your fine motor skills degrade. Fine motor skills are those things that you can't do well when your hands are shaking, like writing, smoothly pressing a trigger, or putting a finger or blade exactly where you want it on a moving target.

Under a more normal dump you lose your complex motor skills. That means your coordination. Anything that involves moving your feet and hands together, for instance. Like combining punches with footwork. Or throwing. Or joint locking. You can still do what you trained, but at a gross degradation in skill.

Under an extreme dump you will either be frozen or drop to a complete passive mode, like a mauled mouse just waiting for the cat to finally kill it. If it offends you that someone you don't know can write about this as if it would affect you, I'm sorry. But you need to know: even heroes die screaming for their mothers. This will affect you if things get bad enough. You can drink your Kool-Aid® of denial and wrap yourself in scrolls and belts and trophies, but those are just talismans to keep the boogey man away. *Even heroes die screaming for their mothers.*

That is just your muscles. Your input process, your senses, change as well. Think about that hard, because if you don't get the information you have trained for you can't make the decisions you have trained for.

Vision gets altered. The most common is tunnel vision, getting extremely sharp focus on a very narrow field. Some reported that they could read their partner's brass as it flew through the air.* That's pretty focused. What it means practically is that you can't see anything coming in from the sides, above, or below. It is very easy to sneak up on people who are adrenalized. I've done it a lot.

Hearing gets downright strange. There is a lot of documentation on auditory exclusion, a very fancy word for temporary and limited deafness. Sometimes you can't hear a gun go off next to your head at all or it sounds like little pops.** You may not be able to hear people

---

* Dr. Alexis Artwohl, "Perceptual and Memory Distortions During Officer-Involved Shootings" *FBI Law Enforcement Bulletin* October, 2002.

** This fascinates me because at least one source in Dr. Artwohl's article mentions not experiencing ringing in his ears after the shots. Which seems to imply that, somehow, the ears physically close-off.

shouting, even when "Behind you!" would be a really useful bit of information.

At the same time, the sound of the Threat breathing may be deafening.

The sensitivity in your hands and fingertips may be completely gone. People drop things under adrenaline, a lot. They can't easily dial phones or work keys. The same mechanism that robs them of their fine motor skills also numbs the fingers. It is good to feel less pain, bad not to be able to feel the body weight or targets on the Threat.

6.1.3: training and you

You have probably heard many times that you will fight the way that you train. It is sort of true. You will fight in this weird mix of the way you trained, your ethics, your instincts, and all of that in a hormone stew. At the best, you will rise to the level of your training, but even that only works if what you have trained against resembles what you are facing. You must know your violence dynamics and train with respect to how predators really attack.

Under attack, you will not have either the mind or the body that you have trained. You will have an impaired, partially deaf and blind, clumsy beginner who isn't that bright. You will be like a rank beginner because, surprise, you are a rank beginner.

Good training will still help because it will work, and that old part of the brain isn't completely stupid. It will go with what works (and then, of course, it will try to turn whatever worked into a talisman and a ritual. Nature of the human beast.) As you make things work, your skills will resurface. Most of what is taught in Self-Defense and Martial Arts work. But you will almost certainly have to make yourself act.

Training that matches the real thing helps. Differences in expectation and reality create glitches. Glitches freeze you. Nothing works every time so you must practice recovering from failure. The Threat chooses the time and place so you must practice working from positions of disadvantage.

This is personal, and one of those things that is good life advice. I don't stretch or warm-up before training. Except for tactical operations I have never had time to warm up before a real fight. As much as possible, I want to train with the body I will have when I fight, old, tired, injured, and stiff as that may be. The reason this is good for life is that stretching and warming up shouldn't be something you do only at class. Life is better when you stretch in the morning, do at least a light warm up and stay stretched and active all day.

Do isometric abdominal workouts when you are driving; stretch your shoulders, spine, and legs in spare moments. Take stairs. Run when you can. Make moving well not just something you do in training but something you do all the time, and something you do in the places and wearing the clothes that you will have to adapt to if things go bad.

6.1.4: mitigating the effects

There are some techniques for dealing with the Survival Stress Response (SSR). Bruce Siddle in *Sharpening the Warrior's Edge*[*] reviews a lot of the literature on the SSR and indexes it to heart rate (note, the heart rate is a *symptom* of the hormone dump, it doesn't cause it). Techniques to lower heart rate are used to lower the level of stress hormones.

The weakness in all of these systems is that they take time. If someone is trying to decapitate you with a machete you don't have *time* to take four calming breaths. Breathing is one of the things you can do during the interview while you are gathering information and looking for a way out. Breathe in to a count of four, hold for a count of four, breathe out for a count of four, hold empty for a count of four; repeat. I use longer counts, but the four count is commonly taught.

Clearing the spine and grounding can also work. Consciously feel the earth with your feet, suck your weight down, feeling gravity. Give your feet a slight twist like you are working them into sand, then let that twist move up to your hips, spine, shoulder, and neck. This has an

---

* Siddle.

added advantage in that I have never had an experienced fighter who saw me clear my spine decide to fight. This can be combined with the autogenic breathing above.

Centering is a psychological first aid technique for children but I've found it very useful for both calming myself and others and concentrating on the moment. Right now, notice and identify five sounds (I hear my son's fork on his plate, the heater humming behind me, bad Irish music playing in the background, chewing, a chair settling under weight) five touches (my forearms across the edge of the table, a breeze across my bare feet, my pulse in the back of my upper left jaw, the hair in my nostrils moving as I breathe, the carpet under my bare feet) and five scents (my son's omelet, apple tobacco in the nargilah, soapy water in the kitchen, my own skin after just waking up, hot dust from the heater). Centering is another of those good life skills. Calming increases your awareness and forces you to focus on senses, particularly scents that your consciousness usually ignores.

Self-talk got me through my first real injury as a medic. You just tell yourself what to do and do it. Let yourself be back in student mode: "I need to fight this guy and I'm getting my ass kicked, what would coach say?" Then be your own coach. I have used this out loud, taking down a Threat while explaining what I was doing and why: "Sir, as long as you keep resisting I'll have to use force. If you don't roll over onto your stomach, I'm going to have to roll you over and if you keep thrashing I'll kneel on your neck and that will hurt a lot." Even when I was actually talking myself through the process, the Threat and all the witnesses interpreted it as giving fatherly advice, trying to not use force. It works that way, too. Sometimes really angry or drugged or drunk people don't know or remember how to give up. Telling them how works fairly often. Also, many people forget to breathe under stress. If you are talking out loud, you are breathing.

The one that takes the least time and the one that I have used most in the midst of an actual fight doesn't actually calm so much as switch modes. It is something I picked up from an off-hand comment from George Mattson, one of the Grand Old Men of karate in the United States. He said, "If you can smell things, you're breathing right." What I found was that consciously smelling the Threat not only kept me breathing but was both calming and put me in a predator mindset.* It was very, very effective.

6.2: the threat(s)

There are lots of differences between the Threat or Threats that you will face in an assault and the partners you train with. First and foremost, Threats are not your friends. You care about the people you train with and they care about you. A Threat does not care if you make it to class next week or not.

This has two huge implications for how you train and the effect that your training can have. Martial arts is *about* breaking people. In every drill that you do, every match, every tournament where you do *not* break your partner a safety flaw has been introduced into the training. You are doing something and have been trained to do something (pulling punches, wearing 16 oz gloves, pulling up on the follow-through to a throw . . .) that is specifically designed NOT to hurt your opponent. This habit has ingrained just as hard as anything else you have trained.

The second implication is that the Threat has not trained this way, so when he hits you or cuts you it will not look and feel like you have trained. Unconsciously, you have counted on the safety flaws and may even rely on them to make your own techniques work. *When you realize those safety flaws are gone you are once again vulnerable to a freeze.*

Threats do not attack like partners. The four things that shock most trained martial artists in their first fight are:

Attacks happen much faster than they train against. In an ambush, the Threat goes for a flurry of damage, not the give and take of sparring. In an all-out assault completely untrained people hit at least four times a second. Well-trained martial artists hit about ten times a

---

* Predator doesn't automatically mean bad guy. When officers make mistakes it isn't because they were thinking coldly, like a predator. It is almost always because they were thinking emotionally, like a monkey, letting their ego and social status concerns influence judgment. For a Criminal Predator, violence is a tool to get something. For a good guy in predator mode violence is a tool to end something quickly, efficiently, and above all, safely—for everybody if possible.

second. That is much, much faster than most people train for. That is why so many people get caught in the Observe-Orient bounce.

Bad guys hit harder than you train against. It shouldn't be *surprising*, but most find that first face hit *shocking*. Whether it is done with a bitch slap or a pitcher of beer, crooks hit hard. It is how they win. Boxers hit hard as well and martial artists certainly can hit hard—but between the gloves and the safety equipment and the safety flaws too often someone striking with intent to injure is an entirely new sensation.

The assault happens at very close range. Martial arts and martial sports universally start their matches just out of range. Closing to contact range is part of the skill. Threats use guile or ambush to cross that range so that when they attack it is fast—distance is time in an assault and close is often too fast to block; it is hard—the attack comes at the optimum range, the Threat doesn't have to reach for anything or sacrifice balance; and it is a surprise. There's no bow-in, no handshake, no ref saying, "Let's get it on!" There is a hit, too fast, too hard, and too close coming from nowhere.

It is a surprise. If the Threat can tell that you expect to be attacked, he can always wait for a different time or a different victim. One of the things about predation versus social violence is that to a predator, who you are is irrelevant. If you want to be a hard target, he can find a soft target. Victims are interchangeable. In scripted drills or sparring matches, martial artists always know when something is coming. Assault victims don't.

Predators attack harder, faster, closer and with more surprise than training partners.

Training partners also tend to smell better and be healthier than Threats in the wild. Poor hygiene, diseases, oozing sores, and blood-born pathogens are just part of the package at certain strata of the criminal society. There is a work safety rule: if it's wet and it's not yours, don't touch it. It's nice but the choice here may be to take a chance on contracting a disease that will change your life drastically and possibly kill you in seven or ten years . . . or to die tonight.

Some Threats will try to use this as a verbal tactic as well: "If I hit you, you can't hit me back. I have AIDS." I explained to him the fallacy of the logic. He chose the wiser course.

Especially if you train in only one system, you have a pretty good idea of the way your opponent will attack. You and your partners have been taught certain ways to punch, kick, or stab. You are used to defending against those attacks. You get in trouble if you believe those are the only ways that attacks happen. I have heard experienced martial artists say, "No one attacks from that close." "No one can do damage standing nose to nose" and "No one ever attacks with a knife overhand in an ice pick grip."

Yeah, they do. And they try to use shopping carts as weapons and will drop a padlock down a sock to use as a bludgeon. They will bite and scratch and try to stab you with used hypodermic needles. They will try to spit their own blood in your face and vomit or even shit themselves to make you afraid to touch them.

You know what to expect in training, what kind of attacks, the number of opponents, whether weapons are involved. You don't know, except for the Monkey Dance, what to expect from a Threat.

The Threat may also not react like a partner. Some are in altered mental states: drunk, drugged, mentally ill, or emotionally disturbed. What you have been taught about pain may well not apply. The Threat may not even notice you grinding a nerve point, might not even flinch when his jaw breaks. Even the things you have been taught as physiological "musts" are not certain. Head and hands may not move toward a pain the Threat doesn't even feel. He might not curl up even with a good groin strike. Some people can fight just fine blind (this is extremely close range, remember, and touch is both more reliable and faster than sight) and your eye-gouge may just piss him off.

That is just the physical stuff. We all have certain expectations of how humans will react to damage. More often than not those expectations spring from psychology, not physiology. We expect someone we shoot in the heart to have the decency to die quickly but there is nothing in a shattered heart to keep a sufficiently dedicated Threat from aiming and firing his own weapon for a full ten seconds. You can be killed by a dead man who simply refuses to acknowledge his own death.

In 1990, Los Angeles Police Department officer Stacy Lim, off duty, was accosted by four men and shot in the chest with a .357 magnum. The bullet damaged her liver, nicked her heart, and destroyed her spleen. She returned fire and chased the primary threat killing him while the others fled. She survived.

We expect pain or fear or a broken bone or exhaustion to make the Threat quit fighting. Usually, but not always. And this has no automatic answer. Hit ten people in the head in the exact same way and one might pass out, three flinch, two not notice, one run, one go into a murderous rage, and one just look at you like you are an idiot. And the last one may laugh because this is fun! You don't know what kind of Threat you are dealing with until you deal . . . and even that may change because if you are winning some will run and some will try to surrender and some will lash out in a panic. The Threat's personality may change in the course of the encounter. Your personality may be changing too.

You have to deal with the Threat that is in front of you and adapt to what you see.

6.3: the environment

Martial arts and martial sports standardize and simplify the environment so that they can better judge and test specific skills. The more variables in a situation the more luck plays a role in deciding the outcome, and luck is the enemy of a contest of skill.

Here is the Law of dealing with the environment:

Whether something is a hazard or a tool depends entirely on who sees and exploits it first.

The world is big and full of many things. Soft footing, slick footing and uneven footing. Obstacles that can trip or shield or take the impact of a well-propelled head. Tools and junk that fit the hand for protection, offense or distraction. Clothing that can act as armor or handhold or blindfold.

Training to use the environment, is one of those things that is infinitely complex. Within reach right now there are dozens of things I can use for weapons, wall configurations that will and won't stop bullets, obstacles I can exploit or move, light and shadow I can use to distract or gather information. It is infinitely simple. What can I use? How?

It is merely a practice at seeing possibilities quickly. That basic.

It's not something I recommend learning in the conventional way, finding a guru who will introduce you to many found weapons that you must memorize. It is a way of thinking, something that you can incorporate in every area of your life.

There are some exercises for it. Here is one: take the first object that comes to hand and come up with twenty uses for it separate from its primary use. I'm typing on a laptop, so using that as my example, I can use it as a:

- Mirror to look behind me (with the power off, the screen acts as a dark mirror);
- Signal mirror;
- Measuring device (I know the size of the screen);
- Tool to estimate elevation;
- Drafting compass (by holding a pen against the hinged lid);
- Method to estimate angles of elevation;
- Press;
- Book end;
- Weight/plumb bob;
- Straight edge;
- Distraction for a restless baby;
- Commodity to barter for something else;
- Fire starter (using the battery, almost for sure);
- Method to determine if a patch of ground is level
- Clipboard
- Very expensive Frisbee®;
- Lid for the jar in which I've captured a bug;
- Paddle for a raft;
- Equipment to condense water, or, of course;
- Weapon to whack someone over the head with.

Those are without taking it apart, except for the battery.

It might be a cheesy example, but it is a great drill. Only a part, though. The habits you developed in the section on escape and evasion are also a big piece of this. That was an introduction in how to look at terrain. One of the keys was recognizing windows and walls that you could break.

Another drill—look at any object and ask yourself, "What is it really?"

I'm typing in a brew pub in Portland on a small table. What is it really? It's a square of solid wood, about twenty-two inches on a side composed of eight tongue-and groove pieces of varying widths (that's odd, it must be quite old). It rests on a single metal post with a four-armed top and bottom, metal, painted black. Probably iron, from the sound. Cast iron? Each of the four upper arms has two screws holding it to the wood. Under each of the four lower arms is a rubber disc to protect the floor.

What is it really? A weight, a composition, a dimension.

What is it really? Whatever I choose to use it or a piece of it for: splinters and weapons and weights and grapnels and anchors and . . .

If you are like most people your eyes slide off a chair the second you name it "chair." It then becomes something to sit in and all the other cool possibilities go away. We do this with chairs and we do this with space, looking for the familiar ("This part of the place is flat and level, like the training hall, I'll try to fight here"), instead of exploiting the cool and unusual.

Lastly, we do it with people too. Once you identify someone as a Threat or an enemy (and that moment is important to recognize) you shut down some other possibilities. Next time you roll with a training partner, just as an experiment instead of thinking of him as a partner or an opponent, think of him as a toy, a great big cat toy. And you are the cat. Play with him.

Or think of him as a tool, see that everything he does is really to help you.

Using the environment is entirely a matter of how you think and see. It all works for you if you figure it out.

6.4: luck

Luck is whatever you don't see coming. All the variables you didn't see or didn't take into account. You can't control it, that's what makes it luck. On a bad day it can outweigh everything. I try to explain sometimes on a tactical operation, an entry, we try to minimize luck. We like to know the layout, where everyone is, whatever we can know about everyone there. Weapons, obstacles. We brainstorm, we practice . . . and then we go in. No matter how well we plan or how good the plan is, there is always a chance that one of the good guys will slip in a tiny puddle of sweat, hit his head and it will be "game over."

Professionals do everything they can to minimize luck but there is no way to eliminate it. Bad stuff happens.

6.4.1: gifts

The universe offers you gifts all the time. The key with luck is to recognize the gift and use it. You can say thank-you later. A fist coming at your head is in general a bad thing. If there is a concrete wall behind your head, a slight shift turns the bad thing into a gift, a Threat who breaks himself.

Cell extractions are a big part of a Corrections Tactical Team's job. You have an inmate who may be armed with shanks (prison-made stabbing knives) or flails (like the padlock in a sock) who covered his windows and probably soaped his floors. Before the days of the Taser, the team was expected to handle this unarmed and not to injure the inmate or get injured. The short version of the technique was to slam the Threat into the wall, whip his legs out from under him so that he landed on his back, lock up his limbs, flip him to his belly and cuff him up.

In training once upon a time I was playing the bad guy and instead of trying to stand and fight or dodge, I dove at the entry team's legs. They were good natural fighters and well-trained. They came down on me like a ton of bricks, face down in the concrete. Then they flipped me over to my back, locked up my joints, and rolled me back over to my front to cuff.

Hmmmm. They had not recognized that my actions had given them the first three steps of their plan. They didn't recognize the gift. We had a long talk and it is still something I emphasize with almost every class: nothing works because you do it well, it all works because the Threat or the world made it happen. Specific locks or take-downs work because the Threat was in the position and giving you the momentum for that particular lock or take-down. You don't get an armbar in real life on someone pulling his arm back . . . but that action of pulling the arm back is THE gift that allows a shoulder or wristlock. Even strikes don't work unless the Threat gives you the gift of an opening.

This is one of those things that I suspect can make your life deeper and richer, but I have trained myself to look for gifts in dangerous times. The opportunities are there always and in all ways, in friendship and romance, in opportunity and new ideas. Every second the universe offers you gifts to make life better, if you learn to see them and accept them.

6.4.2: managing chaos

There is a lot going on in any fight, more stuff than your conscious brain can conceivably manage. When you are winning, you want less stuff going on. When you are losing, you want more.

When winning, minimize chaos; when losing, increase chaos.

Winners must consolidate their position, moving towards winning is moving towards a state of control. This is what "position before submission" is all about. If you have absolute control you can win whenever you choose. As control lessens so does your ability to guarantee a win.

As the target of an assault, you will start with little or no control and you will have to take opportunities as they present or make opportunities. That should be a part of the tactical skills of any martial art or self-defense that you study. Your instructor may not use the same words, but exploiting and creating opportunity are inherent (if not explicitly stated) in all martial arts.

Increasing chaos is subtly different: instead of creating opportunity, you are creating opportunity for opportunity. You are being strangled from behind and the Threat knows what he is doing. You have 7–9 seconds of consciousness. After that, whether you live or die—and how you will die—will be entirely up to the discretion of the Threat.

Getting your feet under you and throwing both of your bodies through a window or down the stairs or into traffic might hurt you more than the Threat. Or it might hurt the Threat more than you. In any case, it will throw variables into the situation. If you are going to lose and possibly die in seven seconds, *something* needs to change. Maximizing chaos is rolling the dice that the change will benefit you. It is not as risky as it might sound for two reasons.

First, you are losing anyway. Like breaking ribs during Cardio Pulmonary Resuscitation, it sounds awful but you can't argue that you made the patient worse than dead. Dead with broken ribs isn't worse than dead, alive with broken ribs is considerably better than dead.

Second, fighting is far more mental than physical. In introducing chaos one advantage lies with you: the Threat has to adapt to a major change that you knew was coming. You may be injured more or not, but almost certainly the Threat will be surprised more. He may freeze or panic or give up a sure win to protect himself from a possible loss (that is what the palm-heel to the face versus the knife thrust does).

6.4.3: discretionary time

Gordon Graham does talks on Risk Management for Law Enforcement agencies. I shamelessly stole this from him but then went around and applied it to fighting, which isn't his thing.

Sometimes you don't have to do anything. If someone were silly enough to grab both of your wrists, so what? Other than a headbutt or a kick, both of which you can do with less telegraph than the Threat, what danger are you in? There are ground fighting positions where the Threat is in a clearly dominant position (in judo he would be declared the winner after holding one for 25 seconds) where he can't injure me without changing the hold . . . so why struggle? Why not rest?

Rest and plan. And communicate.

There are lulls in fights, times of relative safety. If you have a second, take the damn second and do some thinking. Take a few breaths. See about getting help. Try to get the audience on your side ("Could someone please call the police? I don't think I can hold this guy much longer"). Check to make sure that your ego isn't involved, if you are winning why haven't you left and moved to safety? Are you fighting the urge to transition from self-defense to an Educational Beat Down? That is a strong temptation. If other people are involved (this is mainly for cops) are your partners getting excited?

When these moments happen, professionals exploit them fully.

6.5: the fight

A lot has been covered above: differences in you under stress; between the threats and your training partners; how the environment changes things and the role of chaos. This section will be a little more scattered, pointing out some of the details of real violence that training rarely prepares you for.

Someone is trying to kill you. Even if the intent is not lethal, the Threat is trying to deliver as much force as he can to your body. He is not feeding you a technique. He is also not setting up a layered combination in order to create an opening. The Threat is beating you down. Unlike sparring he will not be holding back either to protect you from injury or his fists from injury or to keep his defense up. His defense is that he is doing so much damage to you so fast that you can't think beyond that. This is how an assault works.

It is not suspenseful. It is not fair. One person gets the advantage as early as possible and ruthlessly pushes that advantage until it is over.

People pretend, but you will rarely see this taught in martial arts classes. If someone swings a club at your head full power and you flub the defense in any way, one of two things happen: you get injured badly or the person manages to get control at the last second to protect

A feed is when you give your uke/partner/student something that looks like an attack but is designed so that they get practice working the technique. It is a technique designed to be defeated, to give practice at block and then strike or simultaneous block-and-strike.

But it is not an attack. It is a feed. Training in this way, even sparring starts to be composed of feeds. Not good feeds, the person doesn't want to lose after all, but not attacks either. Attacks are designed to hurt and damage and overwhelm. Offensive moves in sparring, as often as not, are designed to deceive, disconcert or score . . . which are very different things.

An attack designed to injure, hurt and subdue you mentally and physically is completely different than a feed. It is delivered at a different range with a different intent, often at different targets. It is not a game with the halfhearted commitment that makes for such great contests of skill and timing.

When it is an assault, you add the element of surprise and it becomes a flurry of damage with no thought of defense. As different from an attack as an attack is from a feed.

you. Both are problems—severely injured students mean the school disappears. Being able to pull means that the intent and commitment wasn't there to begin with. If the intent was not there, then what the student was training against did not have the same intensity, feel or timing as the real thing. It is especially poisonous if the students and instructor honestly believe that the intent was killing and pulling was a sign of skill.

Fights are not static. Things move. People move. Bear-hugs and headlocks and all that stuff happen sometimes in a fight, but they are transitional actions. You do not get bear-hugged just to be held (except by bouncers). A Threat wraps his big arms around you from behind either to pick you up and shake you (disorienting and intended as an intimidating show of strength) or to drive you into a wall. Maybe to throw you over a balcony. If you practice technique-based defense, will they work if the Threat refuses to stand there? If he is using that headlock to slam you from wall to wall?

It takes skill and practice, but movement is not a bad thing. Movement is momentum and momentum is a gift, a gift that you can exploit.

Not everything is dangerous. This ties into discretionary time, but also the perception gap. Scary is not the same as dangerous and sometimes it takes a lot of skill to see that.

A guy grabs you by the shirt with both hands, balls up his fist in the material and starts screaming in your face . . . OH MY GOD! What do you do? What if he were screaming this:

"Alright you punk, I'm your attacker and I'm going to start by wrapping up both my hands so that I can't use either one and pulling you close so that my ears, throat, nose, knees, groin, and maybe even cervical spine are all in easy reach for you. On top of that, I'm making sure that all the witnesses around here know that I'm an ass and you didn't have any choice, since the one thing grabbing your shirt does do is keep you from leaving! Plus, the only things I can really do from here are a knee, a low kick, a head butt, or to lift you off your feet, all of which you will feel the lead-up with plenty of time! What do you have to say to that, punk?"

He's trying to be intimidating but it is not nearly as dangerous as your first instinct.

Next time you are playing "what-if games" try, "what if I do nothing?" When you are working on escapes, what happens if you don't escape? You will find several where the danger is not in the hold itself and the Threat must actually transition to something else to do injury. That transition may be the vulnerable point. Don't tire yourself out trying to get out of a safe position, even if it is uncomfortable and smells bad.

It is not a contest. You have the instincts of a puppy, especially if you have trained for a long time in something that you love. When I go to the ground with a criminal I have to fight the instinct to revert to tournament judo. I practiced for a long time, I was good at it, and I loved it, especially groundwork. It also triggers an instinct: wrestling is very much how children and puppies establish dominance and bond.

When both your instincts and your martial training are keyed for dominance, it can be very easy to forget that your primary goal is to escape or to neutralize the Threat. Sifu Kevin Jackson asked me about escaping from a ground position. The Threat has fallen with you in a headlock. He is down, on his side. You are in a semi-kneeling position at his back and he has your neck held tightly to his side.

Kevin went over a number of possibilities and asked what I thought. "The Threat took me to the ground and has control of my neck? I'd just slam his head into the concrete. I don't want to wrestle with him." (See Figs. 6-001)

Kevin is a good martial artist. I'll go out on a limb and say that he is an extraordinary martial artist but sometimes that bites him on the ass (and it does it to all of us) when he forgets the difference between training to win a dominance contest and training to survive. All sparring matches—weapons, duels, Mixed Martial Arts, or point fighting, are dominance contests, not survival contests. But they are sure fun.

Fight to the goal. Goals differ in different situations. Generally in self-defense you are fighting to escape. Sometimes you may need to fight to neutralize the Threat if there are other helpless potential

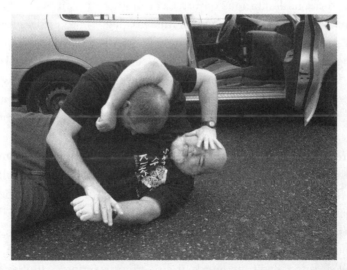

Fig. 6-001: Why do a fancy grappling escape when you can just slam his head into the concrete? Repeat as necessary.

victims who would not be safe if you left. Sometimes getting enough air to yell for help is all that you can do.

What you need to do changes how you fight. Recognize this and, critical in a self-defense situation, recognize when you are reverting to your training goals. No magical ref will appear and award you a win after a three-second pin. The guy may be too unstable to surrender when you get him in your nifty armlock, and if he did surrender, how would you know it was sincere and how would you safely transition to your escape? What if he didn't surrender and you snapped the joint and he just kept fighting like nothing happened?

If the goal is to neutralize the threat, to take him out, it must be a dedicated, explosive effort. In essence, you will have to out-blitz the blitz Predator.

Fights are multi-layered. The four elements: you, the Threat(s), the environment and luck; physical and mental forces; legal and social customs; what the fight is about and what both parties *think* it is about.

The more broadly you can see the situation, the more options you have and the more dangers you can avoid. Being aware of the physical environment gives you tools and allows you to avoid hazards. Recognizing the legal limitations on force can both keep you out of trouble and possibly provide leverage ("Is this worth going to prison, son?").

I strongly encourage most people to keep trying to communicate during the fight. The least it will do is clue in the witnesses. This is most important legally when you are winning. Since the goal was to escape if you are winning and haven't escaped, an explanation will help clarify: "Let me go! I just want to leave! Let go of my arm so I can leave!"

Winning or losing, it can play on the Threat's social conditioning to end things, especially if it was an Status-Seeking Show or Educational

> Your tactics and techniques must serve your strategies and goals. If your strategy is to escape and your primary techniques are locks . . . how does that work?

Beat-Down and the audience is watching, "You win, dude, just let me go." (And this will trigger all of your monkey buttons, it will feel like surrendering or even begging and you have millennia of genetic conditioning not to do it. You will have to decide if you are more man than monkey and do the smart thing, and trade an internal shame for injury.)

You are fighting a mind, not just a body. On the rare occasions when I teach knife defense (and the name of the workshop is "Why I don't pretend to teach knife defense" which tells you something) the first thing we establish is how little actually works against a fast aggressive blade or the common blade assassinations.

In the class I explain that the thing that gives you a chance against weapons or multiple attackers or any situation of extreme disadvantage is to fight the mind. When it is my turn for the guy to come at

On men and women and perceptions of fighting: A lot of the monkey stuff is purely imaginary. Young men don't fight because women will think they are cool. Young men fight because they *imagine* that is what women will think.

An acquaintance walking with his girlfriend in a remote area backed down from a Group Monkey Dance. They had stumbled on a group of about six young men partying on the beach. He backed down and got out of there. And, he was sure the relationship was over, that his girlfriend couldn't possibly be satisfied with a wimp and a coward.

The math was obvious: six on two, young men, remote area, alcohol and drugs. His monkey brain was beating him up for not risking a beating (minimum) and likely a gang-rape for his girlfriend and possible torture murders for both.

I advised him to talk to his girlfriend about it and told him that women did not see these things the way men did.

This thing that had been eating at him for months? She barely remembered it. She had had no thoughts about his courage or manliness whatsoever. She remembered one fleeting thought of being happy with a man who wasn't stupid.

me with the knife I don't block or evade. I hit him. And I scream. The scream is what freezes the Threat and buys the time for technique to work. Sometimes I even pull one hand out of the fight, reaching behind my hip as I scream "Drop the weapon! Do it now!" in my best cop voice. It is amazing the number of students who clearly see the gun, can even describe it in detail, even though my hand was completely empty.

With the exception of lethal force, of actually shutting down the brainstem, you do *not* beat people. They give up. Anything you can do that influences them to give up or encourages them to walk away is good. Anything that jacks them up, that makes them afraid to stop fighting, is bad. Making threats in a fight ("I'm gonna stomp you into jelly") can raise the stakes and make it *harder* for the Threat to quit. Intimidation might prevent a fight but during a fight it becomes incentive to intensify the resistance. If you believed you were going to die would you give up?

Fighting the mind: you can freeze them, psych them, or influence them.

The sudden shout (or sudden, sharp pain) can make the Threat *freeze* for an instant and buy you enough time to do something else. Saying or doing something weird or unexpected can lock him into the Orient stage of his Observe-Orient-Decide-Act loop. Rapid movement, especially combined with rapid speech can force him into the Observe Orient bounce. Re-read the section on freezes, but this time look for how many of them you think you could *induce in the Threat.*

Letting the Threat know that he can't win or putting him into a position where he feels that *he* has stepped through the looking glass influences the Threat to find other options. It psyches them out. I won't go so far as to say I like being hit, but over the years being tagged in the face has become an indicator that the rest of the evening is going to be really fun. I'm actually thinking jujutsu classes with Dave and brawling classes with Mac, but what a Threat sees is someone who likes getting hit. When I get hit I smile and sometimes giggle. That's profoundly not normal. It makes the Threat rethink his choices.

So does maintaining a calm professionalism. This is more a cop thing, but using an emotionless Jack Webb ("Just the facts, ma'am.")

voice in the middle of a fight is extremely disconcerting. "Son, I really don't want to hurt you, but this hurts now and it's going to hurt a lot more. Just let me put handcuffs on you and we're done." Or the pre-assault classic when a criminal challenges me to fight, "Up to you. I get paid whether you go to the hospital or not."

Psyching can also be physical. One of my favorite techniques is to pass an attack and face-mask the Threat, bending his spine backwards but not letting him fall. It is extremely disorienting to be twisted and not even be able to fall. Most (all so far) become very happy to talk.

One more example. The U.S. Marines' manual *Warfighting* advocates war of maneuver. ". . . we see that the aim in maneuver warfare is to render the enemy incapable of resisting by shattering his moral and physical cohesion . . . rather than to destroy him physically . . ." The manual advocates the ability to move and change in space and time in order to create a situation the enemy cannot cope with. Not one the enemy can't win. Not to destroy the enemy, but to overwhelm the enemy's ability to cope. Coping is a mental skill. Beating the mind, not the army.

Influencing relies heavily on Peyton Quinn's advice to leave a face-saving exit. You want him to leave without feeling like he is running. People will fight for their imaginary manhood even when it is stupid, so you never take that away. "The cops are going to be here soon," allows the Threat to avoid jail rather than run from you. "I give up," lets the Threat feel like the winner.

Influencing can work before the fight as a de-escalation technique and occasionally in the moments of discretionary time that occur during the fight.

Fighting isn't all about one thing. In many martial arts you have very limited definitions of winning (throw for ippon, 25-second pin, submission, knockout . . .) and the techniques and tactics you learn are based on that goal. Fighting is more wide open with more possibilities.

If you are trained to go for the knockout, you may miss the gift that sets up a takedown or vise versa. At any moment you can do at least one of four things. You can move (the Threat, a part of the Threat or yourself) cause pain, damage, or shock.

Movement. Sometimes when you can't do damage, you can still push or pull the Threat off-balance; or you can use his head to control his spine; or position one of his limbs so that he can't effectively attack you; or position one of his limbs to expose a target; or move yourself to a place where you can safely get control.

Sometimes you can *cause pain* with a pinch, a slap, or a pressure point. Be aware that pain is idiosyncratic and unreliable. Not everyone feels pain the same way or reacts to pain the same way. When you do use pain it is for one of three reasons—to temporarily freeze the Threat's brain; to draw a specific flinch; or as a bargaining chip ("You quit fighting and back off and I'll let go of your nipple ring").

Damage is anything you do that is intended to make a Threat unable to move a body part or use a sense. People have a tendency to confuse pain and damage. Tasers hurt a lot, but they do no appreciable damage. Getting punched in the nose hurts and bleeds and can make your eyes tear up but it doesn't even slow down an experienced fighter. Many adrenalized fighters do not notice when they break their hands punching, not until later.

Dislocating major joints or breaking long bones are damage. They do not always completely neutralize the Threat, but they make the Threat far less efficient.

Shock is an attempt to shut down the entire system: lethal force, a knockout, a strangle-hold, are all examples of shock. Shock or extreme damage are the only things that will stop a Threat who won't give up. Fortunately, most do give up to fear, pain, or mild damage.

Body blows that cause internal bleeding or that temporarily stop the diaphragm ("knock the wind out") are shock tactics . . . except bleeding out internally can be very slow. When it works it is almost always a psychological reaction to pain, not a physiological shock that stopped the action.

Pain and damage are the natural environments of battle. In sterile training it is easy to forget what you are training for. When self-defense gets physical, it is going to hurt. People will be broken. Joints tear, blood flows. Gravel grinds into skin.

In a class designed to be fun and educational, it is easy to let this simple fact be forgotten.

6.6: a letter to johann—on intervening

This material is edited from a post on my blog. One of the regular readers, Johann, asked: "How would you attack someone from a distance (3m-10m), for example someone busy hurting someone else? No weapons on any side."

"How do you break up a fight?" is a direct question and it merits a direct and effective answer. However, there is a long yet simultaneous processing of facts, observations, nuances, and concerns that elapses between forming this question and reaching the answer it deserves. I'm presenting my response to Johann here not as a technique, but as an example of the complexity present in any encounter.

An incident like this prompted my first blog post in 2005. There was more going on there and I was compelled to write the post because of my exposure to blood during the event, not the incident itself. The other question that weighed at the time was long-term consequences and whether saving a life is always a good act.

So, Johann, I'm going to start with a couple of caveats and general stuff. "No weapons on any side" is an assumption that you cannot afford to make, even in theoretical argument. If you are anywhere in the real world you should be able to access something to use as a weapon even if no one else is doing it. I am more or less expected to take people down without hurting them so sometimes I go hands-on when it might not be wise.

When you are going into a situation it can go bad very, very fast. Be ready for that. Both of the people involved and even the audience might turn on you if they see you as an outsider trying to break up a fight between insiders. If you tunnel-vision on one, you might miss the response of the other. There is a lot that can potentially go wrong.

Have a back-up plan. Preferably have some back-up people who can pull you out if things go wrong. It is a situation that can turn from easy to a 2-on-1 in a heartbeat.

Move fast and decisively. This goes for everything, but if there is any hesitation, any half-assed attempt to do a technique it will fail.

This does NOT mean you try to take heads off! You use the minimum level of force that you believe will work. If you think you can do it with a lock, you do a fast, decisive lock—no hesitation. If you decide you must strike, even try to take a head off, you do it. You don't give a half-power blow to gauge the effect. If you think of the level of force you have chosen as a place, you must be all the way there. If you hesitate at the threshold you will fail.

Johann's instructor recommends going in hard with fists and boots. In my experience, striking is relatively unreliable. I'll go farther than that. The effects can be downright weird. I've seen people curl up in fetal positions from strikes that others ignored and just glare when hit in the head with a bar. Been lifted in the air by a solid groin strike that didn't affect me at all for several minutes and been put down by one that barely contacted. Put people down twice with a solid left hook to the floating ribs but been on the receiving end from bigger, stronger people and didn't feel it. Fought through concussions and not noticed broken ribs.

My experience is that the closer the Threat is to a normal state of consciousness the more likely strikes will work like they are "supposed to," but since the closer one is to the normal state of consciousness the less likely I'll need to go hands-on at all. You do the math. Strikes seem to work best when you need them least.

Those are the warnings. Here is some strategy:

You are not taking damage so you can take a little time to make a plan, or get help, or get a tool. It might sound cold to ignore the person who is taking damage, but this isn't about justice, this is about resources. You do this stupid and get hurt not only do you get hurt, you can no longer be a resource to save the victim. One of the reasons to plan and train for these scenarios is to limit that damage time.

Do it smart. Remember the four basic truths (hard, fast, close, surprise)? Use them. The Threat should have no idea you are there until you have already acted. Fast and hard/decisive action. Part of Johann's question says 3m-10m. Without a weapon, you can't do anything at that range. Part of answering this question is closing the range without being seen. Usually, the Threat is tunnel-visioned and it isn't much of a problem.

Choose which one to help. This sounds stupid but sometimes the guy winning is the good guy. You might not know. This is critical if you are considering deadly force.

Can you fight the mind? In a full-blown berserk rage, probably not. He may not be able to hear you at all and he may not care. Increasing the level of stimulus (trying to distract the Threat) usually increases agitation. That said, there are two strategies that sometimes work:

1) Supplying information, e.g., "The cops are on the way." Or, "You'd better stop; I don't think he's breathing." The more criminal the act is, and by that I mean deliberate and planned and based on a history of successful violence, the more likely these are to work. It's fundamentally fucked-up but career criminals know when and how to surrender. They can keep consequences in mind, like a manslaughter conviction is heavier than an assault conviction, that an enraged citizen or EDP (Emotionally Disturbed Person) couldn't. Remember the line about resources, not justice? This is another part. Stopping someone from being violent isn't about justice, only about cessation.

2) Shocking them. I'm generally soft-spoken but I do have a window-shaking sensei voice. Good thing is that a couple of times it has had almost magical effects on fighters. Bad part is that it ruins my voice for days every time I use it. So we're talkin' really loud noises. I think a bucket of ice water would do wonders (it works on dogs), but I've never been allowed to use it to break up fights with inmates.

Both of these strategies can sacrifice surprise. It's your call.

Take a second now because that is a huge amount of information and we haven't even got to the technique yet. Take that to heart. Technique is the easiest part. Knowing when and how to apply the technique is the second easiest. Making yourself do it may be the hardest and that's the part I'm not sure can really be taught.

All of this gets modified by position. In the example from 2005 the Threat had the other guy bent over backwards on a table, was leaning over him with a forearm choke across his neck and gripping the victim's shirt with his other hand. Had he been in a mount, straddle ground and pound, or clinch it would have changed things.

Coming up on the Threat's right from behind, the left hand goes to control the base of his spine (pelvic girdle) and the right hand held very flat comes up across his mouth and under his nose.

—The spine control assumes he is not laying flat. You only need it if he can move freely from his legs.

—Stay in a position that if he spins suddenly to either side to throw an elbow the elbow will impact something or you can control the rotation at the shoulder before it reaches you.

—Right at the base of the nose is a place where it is still bone and not cartilage. It makes a nice grip, is extremely sensitive to pain and can apply extraordinary leverage through the spine to the whole body.

—Pull up and back with your right hand, and probably push forward with your left.

—Use the bone at the base of your index finger to maximize pain on the nose point.

—The action works on the spine. You don't lift his face you extend and arch his spine. That's why it works on monstrously strong people. (In a lot of techniques, instead of looking for the circle, look for the spiral. If that makes no sense to you, it will in a few years of practice.)

—Pushing forward on the lower spine gives a two-way action (one of the basic principles to making things work) and puts him in a position where he can't generate power in any direction other than falling down.

—Depending on position, but especially if the Threat is now on his feet or knees, you can 'load' the spine a bit by a slightly shifting up and to the left with your right hand.

Be very, very careful with this. Catch me in person to find out why.

Finish. You probably have him in a spine immobilization, which looks like he is doing a back-bend with his hands not touching the floor. I've held people in that position and had chats. It may work and it allows you a chance to keep an eye on the other guy.

You can drop him straight down from there, which may just kick off another ground fight with your back to the other one. You have to keep the other guy in your peripheral vision.

If you have loaded his spine, you can now pivot hard to your right and project the Threat to land face-down. That's what I did with the guy in the example. I was able to do it and keep the other in sight.

I can imagine ways that things could heat up again and leave you in a bad position. My experience is that if it is fast and decisive enough, no one wants to be in the sequel, and this technique looks like magic. We investigate all Uses of Force and this one got some extra hard looks because all of the witnesses said, "Miller showed up and the guy was on the ground." It had happened too fast for the witnesses, including the experienced officers, to tell what happened or how. That's good but it makes the reports look fishy.

CHAPTER 7: AFTER

Rubber bullets are supposed to hurt a lot and bounce off, not tear a hole the size of your thumb into human flesh.

The barricaded Threat who had made weapons and armor for himself looked up and said in a completely dead voice, "Well. Guess I'm gonna have to sue you now."

As soon as the operation ended we could see the Captain pacing back and forth, talking on his cell phone. "This is the worst day of my life," he said.

At the after-action debrief, we checked the munitions and the literature that came with the munitions just as we had done before the operation. It clearly stated the round was supposed to be safe at five feet and I had fired at more than fifteen. I double-checked the data on the company's website where impact data was available at five feet. Within a week the website said that the round was not for use at close range.

No dreams at least. Occasionally a thought would drift out of nowhere, "Hey, I shot a guy." But it didn't feel like that, exactly . . . I'd undoubtedly blown a hole in a human being with a firearm . . . but it definitely wasn't an officer-involved shooting.

Months after the incident everyone involved was cleared by Internal Affairs except for me. Actually, I was cleared. They just forgot to deliver the letter.

Friends drifted away temporarily. It seemed big and harsh at the time but they were just having trouble dealing with an intrusive reality. Training and minor operations could feel like a hobby, like playing a game. Hospitals and gunfire made it a little too real for a time . . .

Win, lose, or draw, if you have to defend yourself and you don't die, you will have to deal with what comes afterward. That can be a lot or a little, depending on you and your preparation, the identity of the threat, the level of force that you used.

There are potential medical repercussions, legal consequences, psychological issues, and sometimes the possibility of retaliation.

Everything you have done in the previous six areas that we discussed will affect how you deal with the aftermath and what aftermath you will be dealing with.

If you decided that training scenarios with respect to the law would pollute your pure and ancient art, you might be looking at manslaughter charges and prison time.

If you never worked out your glitches and froze, you may wake up in the hospital unable to see or speak.

If you never put the time in to study how criminals use knives, you may be in dialysis twice a week until your name finds its way to the top of the kidney donor list.

If you said something stupid, process servers may show up to let you know that you are being sued in civil court for more money than you have ever seen.

7.1: medical

Ideally, your self-defense will never get physical. Avoiding the situation and running or talking your way out – either of these is a higher order of strategy than winning a physical battle. If it goes physical, however, it will not end with all parties unscathed. Someone will be hurt. Maybe everyone. It might be bad.

How bad? You might be dead. Or dying alone in the rain. Or crippled. You might bleed-out slowly in great pain, looking at white chunks on the ground that your blurred vision can't quite resolve into your own teeth.

Too poetic, that last. It is dirty and hurts and you might not win. Even if you do win by some definition, you might die.

There is potential for immediate, medium, and long-term medical effects of violence.

7.1.1: as soon as you are safe

Immediately after you know you are safe, check yourself for injuries. Look at everything you can look at and touch what you can't see. Check your hands for blood after each touch. Feel for pain and for what won't move properly.

Then check anyone else who was involved. Then check the Threat. I heartily recommend first aid classes for everybody. If you have no training you are looking for:

Consciousness. If someone is conscious, his heart is beating and he is breathing. If help is several minutes away, re-check consciousness every few minutes and let emergency medical responders know of any changes.

Breathing. The actual first aid protocol is Airway before Breathing (hence ABC for Airway, Breathing, Circulation) but checking, much less clearing, an airway without endangering the spine is a skill. You can check breathing without touching.

Circulation. If the person is not breathing, feel for a pulse. The carotid pulse on the neck is easier to find than the radial pulse in the wrist.

Lots of blood.

Things that don't look right (e.g., blue lips or heads with big dents in them or arms bent a funny way or bones sticking out of skin).

Do not move any injured people. Unless you have been trained to do an examination, don't touch any injured person.

Immediately call Emergency Services (911) and tell the dispatcher exactly what you see. If you caused the injuries, do not say what caused it or what you did. If pressed, say that they attacked you (and that had better be true or I don't want you reading my book). This is a recorded conversation that will come up in court. Don't say anything that could remotely be construed as incriminating. That said, if the situation is still dangerous, e.g., you drove off the home invasion rapist but do not know where he is at this second, make sure *that* information gets to dispatch. Officers need to know if there still might be a bad guy in the area, particularly an armed bad guy.

Administer first aid to yourself first. If you bleed-out, you can't help anyone else.

7.1.2: hours to months

If there is any concern whatsoever, go to the hospital and get yourself checked. Concussions are tricky and there are lots of different flavors. My first serious concussion felt like I was drunk and hung-over at the same time: nausea and a headache, yeah, but also happy and dizzy and uninhibited. For almost a week. That is not a good sign no matter how it felt.

In a scarier concussion, many years later, I lost consciousness for a few seconds and then passed out twice more in the next two hours. Very bad. Another felt like an ice pick was jammed in my ear. (Never go diving with even a mild concussion.)

If you get sweaty and feel cold or agitated, you could be bleeding internally. There is something disconcerting about pissing blood or spitting blood up after someone tries to strangle you.

While you are being checked-out, talk to the doctor or Physicians Assistant about Blood-Borne Pathogens (BBPs). People have a tendency to bleed in a fight and blood splashes and flows. If knuckles contacted teeth there will be blood contamination (and probably a really nasty infection); or if you bit someone, if blood splashed into your eyes or mouth or into an open wound. There are so many other ways. Threats are members of a criminal subculture. They are at high risk for BBPs, particularly hepatitis. If they don't use needle drugs themselves, someone in their pool of potential sexual partners or previous victims did. Count on it.

A blood test will not immediately show whether you were infected. It can take 2-12 weeks for newly HIV-infected blood to reach a level where the virus is detectable. Parts of your life may be on hold for some time. It is nerve-wracking.

If the Threat was arrested, you can ask that he be tested. If the Threat was contagious, it will be detectable in him. Testing is a medical procedure and it is against the law to force anyone to take a blood test without consent . . . but many officers are very good at talking arrestees into agreeing to a simple blood test. Without consent, it requires a court order, which is both time-consuming and unlikely to go through unless there is an evidentiary need—and the results wouldn't necessarily be shared with the victim, anyway.

Early knowledge is important because there is an anti-viral concoction that prevents HIV infection if it is taken early enough . . . but it has particularly unpleasant side-effects. If you don't need it, you shouldn't take it. If you do need it, you should start it immediately. The trick is in knowing.

For the next twenty-four hours (at least) after a fight, drink lots of water. Water helps to metabolize the stress hormones that built up in your system. Avoid alcohol for the next few days. Alcohol interferes with deep sleep and sleep is where your subconscious will begin processing what happened (again, physical health links to mental health).

The medium-term problems last longer than the day or week. There are some injuries that will take a lot of time, physical therapy, and maybe surgery to get over.

There are others that don't ever offer full recovery but they won't impair your life drastically. My left leg will always be a little bit tight because I had the surgeon use a piece of my own hamstring to repair the ACL. My elbow pops out sometimes, but I can pop it back in. The shoulders grind and there is a constant low-level pain in the right shoulder. My hands go numb if my elbows go above my shoulder . . . that's not a whine. That is just a partial list of part of the price I paid

Be prepared: One of the more common and interesting after-effects of a big adrenaline rush is an almost frantic desire to get laid. The "OH MY GOD I'm still alive" sex can be pretty intense. Other possibilities are the shakes, right after the event; or a very warm, comfortable lethargic feeling. I have seen people who have just given a heroic effort collapse like a marionette with cut strings when it ended. One officer asked if it was normal that he thought he was going to puke and wanted to cry. That's perfectly normal.

in my twenties and thirties to get to my forties. A lot of those injuries happened in training, too. If you are going to play hard, you have to train hard.

If a doctor recommends surgery, get all the information you can about the surgery he recommends as well as other options. Talk to people who have experienced that injury and talk to people who know the surgeon. A friend of a friend at the hospital who knows which surgeons are good and which are . . . inconsistent . . . can save you a lot of pain. If you talk to someone who has gone through the same surgery, he may drop a little tidbit of information like, "I had mine four years ago and it never has stopped hurting." Listen to what those who avoided surgery thought of the choice they'd made, "I avoided ACL surgery on my partial tear through 6 months of couch-sitting, but in hindsight it wasn't worth losing those months." And finally, always get a second opinion before you have an operation. Medicine is the last place where you want to take the path of least resistance.

Go to physical therapy if it is recommended. It will hurt. A lot. The physical therapist's job is to get you better despite your whining and crying. There is often a hefty price to pay for full mobility. You pay that price in sweat and pain. There are no discounts. If you run from the pain, you give up on the recovery.

7.1.3: long-term

I'm completely unqualified to write about this. Combat isn't just about life and death. Being crippled or blind or shitting into a colostomy bag for the rest of your life are all on the table.

I've never been in that situation. I hope to never be in that situation. There are people who have and have gone on to live good lives, read *Gimp* by Mark Zupan—but it isn't the same as the life they knew. It is a jump through yet another looking glass.

If you are in this situation or get there in some future, I wish I could help, but anything I write would be guessing.

7.2: legal aftermath

There are two potential ways that your life can get legally complicated if you use force to defend yourself: criminally and civilly. A criminal process (police, prosecutor, judge and jury, prison) will determine if what you did was a crime, and if and how you should be punished by society. The civil process (plaintiff, lawyers, judge and jury, settlements and findings) operates if an individual or group thinks that you have hurt them and owe them money.

All of my direct experience with these processes comes as an officer working "under color of authority." When it is your job, mandated by society, to get involved in these incidents the rules must be different. Referees don't follow the same rules as players. I'll try to write this from a citizen's point of view with some insider insight.

7.2.1: criminal aftermath

Officers show up at the scene. One or more people are hurt. Others are less hurt. There may or may not be witnesses.

When the officers show up they probably won't have a lot of information. The limited information they do have will color their perception. If the call is "fight in a bar," a couple officers may show up and Oleoresin Capsicum (pepper spray) will probably be the tool of choice. It works on groups. If the dispatcher adds, "weapons involved" more officers will go in with weapons ready and be a great deal more nervous.

The first officers to arrive on the scene don't know exactly what happened or how much danger they are in and they definitely don't know who the good guys and bad guys are. Most are good at reading a scene quickly, but most are experienced enough to know how effective a predator assault can be. If you are the last man standing, a betting man would say that you started it. You start the encounter with the police as the winner presumed to be guilty.

That said, should you even be there? Should you leave before the police arrive? Ideally, you should leave as soon as it is safe to do so because you are going to safety. You do not leave to avoid legal entanglements. That's what criminals do.

Here's a hard truth: criminals are very good at getting away with things. It is part of their job description. If you were to follow the criminal playbook you would get out of there, arrange for some friends to have seen you in another part of town about the same time as the altercation, deny everything and never ever talk to the police. That's what a criminal would do. That combines with another hard truth, or maybe an ethical slippery slope.

If you haven't done anything wrong, the criminal's policy will work too, if you're thinking of using it. Even if it is a pure and perfect case of self-defense, there is an element of luck to the judicial system. Following the criminal playbook minimizes that luck. But it raises the stakes. Fleeing the scene and acting guilty is a strong argument against self-defense. If it fails (and both you and your friends will not be as adept at lying to officers as people for whom that is a way of life) you will fall hard.

This matters because cops are not used to dealing with innocent people. Criminals lie and manipulate, often by acting innocent. They may act innocent more convincingly than you can *be* innocent. Anything you feel like saying or doing as an innocent man will look exactly like the last ten criminals the officer handled who were only trying to *act* innocent.

I am going to advise you to stand on certain rights, e.g., not to talk without a lawyer present. Not only is that what a savvy criminal will do, which makes you look guilty, the officers will play on that perception ("Oh, you need to hide behind a lawyer, huh? So you must have done something wrong."). The officer will then stay silent hoping you will blab all over yourself to fight his perception that you did something wrong. Resist the urge to make-nice and be quiet until you have legal representation.

The officers who arrive on the scene may cuff you immediately. They may cuff everybody. This doesn't necessarily mean that you are under arrest, it is a safety measure. If you see injured people and don't know how it happened it makes sense to deny Means to anyone who may have caused it until things calm down and you have a better idea of what happened.

Miranda rights are one of those things that everyone knows from television and they mostly know it wrong. Do you have a right to have a lawyer present? Yes, if and only if you are 1) under arrest and 2) being questioned. If you are being interviewed by an officer in the street or voluntarily go to the station to answer some questions, you are not under arrest. Miranda does not apply. If you are under arrest and no one asks you a question, anything you choose to say are "spontaneous statements" and fully admissible.

Many officers read the Miranda Rights card to cover themselves, but they are not required to read them and they do not apply unless the person is both under arrest *and* being questioned about the crime.

Then the officers will be asking questions. They will ask you and ask the witnesses. If you're in the right, if you did everything you could to avoid the situation, let the witnesses tell the story.

The officers will ask you what happened. The smart thing to do is to say that you're still in shock and you really want to talk to (your wife, significant other, counselor, pastor) and then call that person and advise them to get your lawyer. If you are extremely confident in your actions and your articulation, you can tell the officer what happened making sure that you cover Intent, Means, Opportunity, and Preclusion and why what you did was the least force that could have worked.

There's a reason I didn't call that the smart choice. It is fine for a professional. *You* will be full of hormones and emotion. Especially if you have severely injured or killed someone, you will have severe guilt issues no matter how necessary it was. Your memory will actually improve after twenty-four hours. What you say in the fog of fear and uncertainty and possibly rage may be wildly inaccurate. Between the bad memory, the guilt, and the after-effects of the Survival Stress Response, you may make inaccurate, even incriminating statements. You may say how sorry you are. You may vent a rage that is really just a reaction to fear. All of your statements can be used by the police and used by civil attorneys in a lawsuit later.

The smart thing is to say nothing until you have talked to a lawyer, preferably an attorney who has expertise in defending self-defense cases.

Do not argue with the officers. If they give an order, obey it. Show your hands, allow yourself to be cuffed. You will probably be coming down from your adrenaline high, feeling a warm sleepy glow. They are just entering theirs. Never force an officer, especially an adrenalized officer, to make a fast decision.

If you are arrested, you will be handcuffed and either taken to a police station for interrogation and then to jail for booking or directly to jail. If placed under arrest, stop talking. At that point say nothing about what happened without legal counsel. Get a competent attorney who knows how to defend innocent people. The public defenders can be good but often they are so overloaded with cases that their priority has shifted from protecting individual clients to time management. If you must use a public defender you will have to be a strong advocate for your position. The attorney is the expert but he or she works for you. You, not the attorney, will be facing jail time.

It will be expensive. One expert estimates that the total court costs for a successful defense of a *lawful* shooting is approximately $50,000. That's a lot of coin but you have to compare it with what you will lose by spending years in prison and having to put "convict" on your job applications.

Either directly from the scene of the incident or after an interrogation at the precinct house, you will be brought to jail for booking. This is more likely for a minor charge if you have *no* criminal record. There is no such thing in the officer's mind as "no record." If you do not have one, you will be taken for positive identification and to have your prints run through AFIS, the Automated Fingerprint Identification System, to make sure that you do not have a criminal record and are not wanted in a different state by another name.

Do not lie about your identity at booking or to the officers. It is an additional charge, usually a misdemeanor, "Supplying False Information." It also will create issues for you in the future, in that as far as the criminal justice system goes, the name you give them may become your "real" name. It will show up as an alias on any background check later.

It also makes it hard to present yourself as a good upstanding citizen just defending one's self when you testify in court.

At jail they will initially take your personal property including money and jewelry. Even your wedding ring. Don't fight them for it. The Corrections Officers don't have a choice. If you are put in a group holding cell and some freak is willing to bite off a finger for something shiny the officers will get blamed. Their fear of liability means that you will have no choice.

Your belt and shoelaces are taken (to discourage suicides). You get a receipt. In my experience the officers are about as polite to you as you are to them. If you get indignant and demanding, they will tell you what to do and they will make you do it. Same if you get whiny and demanding. The booking officers are allowed to use force to get you through the process and they tend to be experts at it: a booking officer will have more hand-to-hand fights in two years than most road officers will have in a twenty-five year career. Do not fight. Be polite. Answer all their questions ("Do you have any weapons or drugs on you, sir? Anything sharp? Where were you born?") that are not about your case, which they probably won't be.

If no one died, you will have a bail amount set. (Murder and treason are two exceptions to the right to bail and most bail amounts are set by statute, though officers can request and judges can approve an increase in bail.) Bail is the amount of money you will owe if you don't show up for court. Bond is about 10% of the bail and is the amount you pay to be released pending trial.

You also may be interviewed by Recognizance (recog) who will determine if you can be "released to your own recognizance" in other words, "let out of jail without paying bond on a promise to appear in court." The recog decision is made based on the seriousness of the crime, your prior criminal history, your ties to the community (living where you were arrested, holding a steady job, two reasons you might not run) and *your attitude*. Never be rude to the recog staff.

If you are a good person, you will likely get "recogged" (released on your own recognizance) unless the charge is very severe, e.g., unless someone died or you used a deadly weapon.* If you are not released and can't make bail you will be held for arraignment. Arraignment is the process of being formally read your charges in a court. A judge is present. It is very common for charges to be dropped at this stage.

If the process goes forward the District Attorney (prosecutor) will take the time necessary to build a case. Your attorney will work on your defense (if you can do anything to help here, legal research or finding contact information for witnesses it can both keep you busy and save you money). Most likely, you will be offered one or more deals. These are offers of reduced charges or lesser penalties in exchange for a guilty plea.

The deals are driven by economics: prisons are crowded and expensive, parole, and probation are much cheaper; trials are time consuming and expensive; courts are crowded, without enough time or space for all the potential cases; the prosecutor's effectiveness is judged by how many cases are closed, not how many are won at trial.

From your end, the deal is about your aversion to risk. Your innocence is not assured, not proven. Trials carry the potential for very hefty penalties. Many states have mandatory minimums for certain violent crimes and if a self-defense case goes to trial it will be as a person-to-person crime of violence.

Reality check and something many martial artists lose sight of: *martial artists are practicing and training in person-to-person violence. As a hobby, they practice and play at things that are heinous crimes except in very narrow circumstances*. The deal will be structured as a risk decision: "Son, if this goes to trial, you could be looking at twenty years in a state prison. But this is your first offense and I'm willing to cut you a deal, two years prison and five years probation. With good time and work time you could be out in fourteen months.**"

---

* A reminder: this whole jail scenario is based on the arresting officers actually making an arrest at the scene. If the witnesses or circumstances confirm self-defense and/or the injuries were minor, they will probably defer an arrest until further investigation or not make one. You will have plenty of time to call your attorney.

** 'Good Time' is time deducted from your sentence for not getting in trouble while incarcerated. 'Work time' is time off for holding down a job while in custody. Together they can reduce time served by about 50%, depending on jurisdiction. In case you were curious why people sentenced to twenty years can sometimes commit another murder 12 years after the first.

Discuss any deal with your attorney but keep some things in mind. Most importantly, a guilty plea goes on your record as a conviction. Even if you get no jail time, every background check from then on will turn up the conviction. Certain career paths will be closed to you. Keep in mind that prison time is not the only penalty of a conviction when you weigh your options.

If an arrest is made, if the charges aren't dropped, if the DA feels the case can be made and if you refuse a deal, there will be a trial.

You will have a choice of a judge or jury trial. If the absolute facts of the case clearly show that you are innocent, go with the judge. However, if the absolute facts showed you were clearly innocent the case would have been dropped. Listen to your attorney. (I say this a lot. Attorneys are pros. Most of what I know about the legal system I learned from criminals and the rest from cops. My view is slightly skewed.)

It will be right here where your preparation from Section 1 will pay off. How well you do in trial will be based on the legality of the

---

Just because you believe, even know in your heart that you are innocent does not mean you are. In a Monkey Dance, Bobby stares. The other guy, Lyle, thinks, *He's starting something.* So Lyle says, "What you lookin' at?"

Bobby thinks, *Jerk's trying to pick a fight? He's starting something.*

We'll skip the next few steps of the MD and get right to the good stuff. Bobby pushes Lyle. Lyle swings. Lyle is a hundred percent certain that he is defending himself because Bobby put hands on first. Bobby is a hundred percent certain that he is defending himself, because Lyle threw the first punch.

Who is innocent? Neither. We can choose to assign more blame to one than the other but neither is innocent. Both played the game.

Not just MD, either. Remember criminal rationalization? You do it too, and you do it with everything you've got when you make a life-shattering mistake. You will come to believe your rationalizations in order to protect your identity, your belief that you are one of the good guys.

You are not the best judge of your own innocence.

decision that you made, whether you executed the decision properly (most of the time meaning that you stopped when it was safe without throwing a few extra strikes in to teach a lesson or "just to be sure") and how well you can explain it. One of the most difficult things is that you must be able to explain the things that happened on the other side of the looking glass to people who believe that the world they live in is the only world.

It's a challenge but what you must explain is: how you knew you were in danger; how much danger you believed you were in and why; everything else you tried and why it didn't work; the things you thought about but didn't try and why (right here is where you make it clear that you also rejected higher levels of force than you used, that the force you did use was what you believed to be the minimum safe level); and, most importantly, why you had no other options. Always explain the reason why to the jury. They need to see how you think, see that in the same situation, they too would have felt there was no other choice.

Never be afraid to talk about your fear on the stand. Fear is the primal justification for defending yourself. Most of the jury may never have defended themselves, may know nothing about fighting that they didn't learn from TV. But they will all understand fear.

7.2.2: civil

The worst of the worst situations and it ends as well as it could: a home invasion robber comes in with a shotgun. Your children are at home. He tells you what he will do to you and your children. He tells you to get the money and credit cards from your purse. He doesn't know you carry a .38 revolver in there. Just for a second a barking dog distracts the invader. You empty the revolver. He goes down still clawing for the shotgun. You call 911.

The police are impressed. It's a Castle Law state and they know that this was a very bad man, so no charges. They give you a card for counseling and say they will be in touch. It is hours before they are done taking pictures and asking questions and take the body away.

The big brown bloodstain will never come out of the rug. You don't know why a stupid stain would trigger the tears.

So it's not all good. Counseling is a good idea and it helps a little with the dreams. Gives you a little insight on why your friends now pull away. The emotions come in waves.

Then a man comes to your door or to your place of work, or you get a registered letter that requires you to sign. It can be up to three years after the shooting. The home invader's mother is suing you, for inflicting deliberate injury, pain, and great bodily harm to the Threat; emotional pain to the mother and the loss of the home invasion robber's potential future earnings.

Not being charged, or even being determined "not guilty" in criminal court is no defense in civil court. Civil court is not an action by the state, so it is not impacted by double jeopardy.

7.2.2.1: the threatening letter

Sometimes all you get is the letter, usually demanding an astronomical sum, and a note to call. If you call, the attorney at the other end of the line will say, "We can make this go away for . . ." he will then name a much lower sum. If a criminal did this it would be called a shakedown, pure and simple. Put you in fear of losing your home, savings, and retirement account and then offer a much cheaper way out. The plaintiff (the Threat's mother in this example) and the attorney both make a little money for just the effort of writing a scary letter.

Sometimes it makes good economic sense. If they are asking for $5,000 and it will cost you more than that in time lost from work and attorney fees to fight it, many people believe the smart thing to do is to pay. Maybe argue them down some more, but pay. It still strikes me as wrong, however, a way for a criminal to continue to victimize someone even from jail or the grave.*

---

* Some inmates sue for fun. As one explained, "It don't cost me nothing, it's legal mail so I don't even pay for the stamps. I got nothing else to do and sometimes they send me money."

> Check your homeowner's insurance policy to see whether it covers claims arising from your acts of self-defense.

Even if you are considering paying, talk to your lawyer and insurance company first. This is thinly disguised blackmail and it may have legal implications. It is possible that if you do pay, without the right contracts and assurances, you can get another letter from another relative later. This is attorney stuff.

7.2.2.2: difference

There are a few differences between the criminal and civil process. In the civil, it is citizen against citizen, not state against citizen. The founding fathers recognized the huge imbalance in power between a private citizen and the state and slanted the rules in criminal court to favor the citizen/defendant. The playing field is more even in civil court and that is a disadvantage to the defendant.

The burden of proof does not rest entirely on the plaintiff. It is not a question of guilt or innocent but of responsibility, and the burden of proof standard is far lower.

In a criminal case (with the exception of affirmative defenses), the burden of proof rests entirely with the prosecutor. The defense could choose to offer no witnesses, not cross-examine, and only say in closing, "You didn't prove anything," and prevail.

In a civil case both sides have to present their version of the events and their interpretations. Facts are important, but emotions are also considered (hence "emotional suffering"). I'm really fighting the urge to say that it is easier for the plaintiff to lie in a civil court. Not exactly, the plaintiff is still under oath, but the plaintiff can present an opinion as fact in ways that a prosecutor never could.

A prosecutor could never simply say, "This was a very bad man." She would have to bring up and prove specific incidents of violence and depravity and leave it to the jury to conclude that the Threat was, indeed a bad man.

In a civil trial, a plaintiff can say, "He was such a good boy. He had some trouble for a while, sure, but he was turning his life around.

He was so loving, so gentle . . ." all about a multiple murderer or serial rapist. And it will stand, not rebutted unless the defendant rebuts it.

Guilt/Not Guilty is a binary decision. In a criminal court there are no "kind of guilty." If a defendant is charged with eight crimes, he or she might be found guilty of six and not guilty on two, but won't be considered 75% guilty. In a civil trial, once it is established that harm was done (if someone was killed, injured or merely lost days of work, some measurable harm was done) the court will seek to show who was responsible for how much of that damage. Here is something you just read but with a slight modification:

It's a challenge, but what you must explain is: how you knew you were in danger; how much danger you believed you were in and why; everything else you tried and why it didn't work; the things you thought about but didn't try and why (right here is where you make it clear that you also rejected higher levels of force than you used, that the force you did use was what you believed to be the minimum safe level); and most importantly, *why the Threat left you no other options*.

You must show in the civil court that the Threat created the need for force, that he refused to let you get out of it, and that he would not let a lower level of force work.

In the home invasion example, the armed Threat broke into the home, the homeowner didn't drag him in. The Threat created the situation 100%. The homeowner could not leave her kids alone with the threat even if she could outrun a shotgun. The Threat took leaving off the table. Coming to the crime bigger, stronger, and armed with a shotgun, the Threat did not leave any options for lower levels of force to work—hitting him with a chair could not have stopped him from pulling a trigger. Neither could wrestling. Even shooting with a handgun wouldn't reliably put him down before he could return fire with the shotgun, it was just the best option the homeowner had.

Not only did the Threat create the situation, but he precluded all other options *by his own actions*. That is what you need to show in civil court.

The standard of proof in criminal proceedings is "proof beyond a reasonable doubt." Ideally, there is no explanation left (excepting magic, aliens, or psychic powers) other than the defendant did it. In civil court, the jury must merely find it "more likely than not," 51% in other words, that the defendant is responsible. This is a side-effect of the "citizen versus citizen level playing field" idea. This makes it critical for you to have an aggressive defense and actively prove that the Threat was culpable.

A last note on the entire legal process. It can take years to settle these things and the waiting can be emotionally crippling. Wondering for three years if you are going to be sued (after the shooting I asked myself almost daily for 1,100 days if today would be the day I would get the notice). Knowing that you had no choice in what you did but may be punished anyway. Hearing someone who did or threatened to do truly horrific things described by his family and friends as "kind" and "loving." The sheer expense and the worry about a complete financial disaster. It's all rough and adds a lot to the psychological pressure.

Making things much worse, anything you say in those three years (except to your spouse, attorney, religious guide, or doctor) could be used against you in a civil suit. When you have the strongest emotional need to talk, it is least legally prudent to do it.

7.3: psychological aftermath

There are a lot of things that you have learned about the world and yourself that are simply not true. Television has told you repeatedly that if you are the good guy everything will be okay in the end. You have probably learned that the world is a relatively safe place because most of it is. You have an idea of how you will handle adversity and danger and fear and pain.

Win or lose, there are usually personal and mental consequences. Survivors of violent encounters may have prevailed, by every measure they may be winners. Or they might be pure victims only alive through luck or the boredom or inattention of their attackers. Sometimes "winners" and victims will have different problems, maybe. But on some days victims feel like winners because they lived and "winners" feel like victims.

If you ever need the information in this chapter, use what you can use. If I use the label of victim or survivor or whatever and you feel you don't fit the label but the rest sounds right, use it. It is yours. You are in charge of your own growth and healing. Just as you should never take the word of a self-defense expert over your own experience, it is doubly true for a stranger who wants to fix your mind. You are responsible to know your own heart and mind.

7.3.1: story telling

Many of the things that you believe right now won't survive that first trip through the looking glass. If you only ever make one trip, if you only have one exposure to extreme violence it seems that all that is left are doubts, things you were wrong about. Sometimes they are not replaced with new truths. In typical human fashion you will make up a new story to replace the old stories. It might be truer. It might not.

I think of humans as storytellers, but stories as well. Every person is a story; his or her identity is something that the person has been creating and reciting, internally, always.

Stories require drama and drama requires conflict. "Everybody got along from the first day to the last," isn't a story. It would be damn boring to watch as a film. Stories should be more interesting than real life. Character in a story is shown in how the person deals with conflict. So our own character our own story, the ones we make up in our heads, are heavily influenced by conflict. If we have experienced little conflict or low-level conflict, it doesn't matter. The character in our head has been fighting dinosaurs and black knights since childhood.

When the rubber hits the road our imaginary white knight or imaginary morally superior pacifist is sometimes shattered in pain and humiliation, but bodies are usually good at healing, eventually. The damage done to this imaginary idea of who we are can be shattered irrevocably.

That's only part of it because there can be a psychological cost even if it goes well. "Othering" is a form of mental gymnastics, and even though the Predator may have skill and experience and has "othered" you completely, it is unlikely that you have fully "othered" him.

187

Some criminals can walk away and get a good night's rest after beating, raping or killing a mark. If you defend yourself and take a life, you will likely see the Threat, no matter how depraved, as a person. It is a courtesy he would not extend to you (if he did he could not make his life through violent crime). It is one of those things that hurts and can feel like weakness even though it is a strength.

By fully seeing what you have done and what it meant, you can learn and understand on a level that a Predator is literally incapable.

If you have studied martial arts for years you may still be beaten, robbed, raped—and you will feel betrayed. Part of the story in your head revolved around using your skills to serve and save and protect. It is a painful thing to fail.

But strangely, if you have studied for years and your skills work exactly the way they are supposed to, that may be shocking as well. One man, suddenly confronted by a bad guy with a knife, moved twice. He did exactly what he was trained to do. He shattered the Threat's arm and did so much internal damage that the doctors were not confident the Threat would survive surgery. The martial artist who defended himself was devastated. Nowhere in the years of practice and visualizing opponents had the messy part of shattering bones and rupturing organs, the loud pops and little wheezy screams, made it into the story.

The enlightened thing to do of course is to abandon the story. Decide who you are when it is appropriate and discover who you are the rest of the time. Easier said than done.

Who you *really* are is fluid and changeable. If not, there would be no such thing as moods. People wouldn't change or learn as they age. Dehydration wouldn't make us agitated and sleep deprivation wouldn't make us irritable. We know these things about ourselves, about our moods. Isn't it insane to realize that we have different personalities on too much caffeine and then expect to be our same old selves when we are terrified?

7.3.2: change

IT IS OKAY TO BE OKAY.

Someone needs to say that and, if you are a survivor (whether of crime or war or a bad childhood) you need to hear it. It is okay to be okay. When people all around you are telling you how tragic it was, how devastated you must be, and what horrible psychological problems you are going to have, you start *expecting* to be damaged. Then you become damaged. Because that is the story everyone is telling you, it becomes the story you tell yourself.

It will probably hurt. Change hurts. But you have been through big changes before. Unless you are crippled or brain-damaged, even an extremely violent crime does not have the physical and neurological impact of, say, puberty. Puberty involved huge physical changes, hormonal changes, status changes, and a major re-wiring of your brain.

Puberty wasn't as traumatic, after a while, because you always expected to grow up some day. Always knew that the man or woman you would become was *supposed* to be different than the child you were.

Surviving violence doesn't change your body like puberty. The hormones from the attack will wash out of your system. Violence *can* rewire parts of your brain for flinching and hyper-vigilance. All minor compared to puberty.

The destructive psychological power of violence is in the damage to your imaginary, constructed, fantasy identity.

So, I'm telling you now if you can use it, expect to be changed. Just like puberty. Maybe less, because you are smarter now. You *will* be changed and that is entirely natural. Don't let anyone tell you that what you are feeling is wrong (don't always act on the feelings, especially the rage and the gibbering terror, but don't ever be ashamed to feel them). Here's a big clue: you lived. The person giving you advice and all the others in the same circumstances might have taken their own ill-considered, ill-informed, patronizing advice and wound up dead or babbling idiots. *You survived.*

You survived the event and you will survive the aftermath.* Do not let anyone tell you there is something wrong with adapting.

Once on a graveyard overtime I brought a cup of good coffee to one of the deputies and we talked. I was going through some rough times, a cumulative mass of big events that wasn't settling like it should. He was going through rougher times. We sat for hours, talking, surrounded by sleeping inmates. It was honest talk about loss and change and toying with the idea of suicide. Finally he said, "Sarge, no one commits suicide because of what happened to 'em. They commit suicide because they thought about it too much."

So . . . we cut down on the thinking about stuff. We've both kept moving since then, kept active. If there is one piece of advice I can give a survivor it is this: when given a choice between agonizing on the past and living, live. Live the life you have and live it hard. Go fishing. Hug your kids. Workout. Hike. Read, even.

You are still you, the only thing you lost was a story that was never true anyway.

7.3.3: feelings

Just so you know, there is no way you can feel about the event that will feel right or comfortable. If you are elated (the battle joy is very real) during or after, you will feel guilty and think there is something wrong with you. If you feel guilty, you will berate yourself for the stupidity of feeling guilty when you had no choice (or possibly worse, you will work to find some details to make the guilty feeling "right"). If you feel nothing, you will wonder what kind of a monster you might be.

There is no right way to feel about an event that wasn't "right" by any normal frame of reference. Just acknowledge how you feel to yourself, perhaps to a few close friends. The general public doesn't need to know about the battle-joy or rage. It's none of their business anyway. Acknowledge your feelings and do not try to justify them.

---

* Because I said so. Seriously. Take a breath. Feel that? That's being alive. That means you won. You survived. The only thing that can kill you now is you. Just don't destroy yourself. How hard is that?

That is a whirlpool that leads nowhere. Emotions are reactions from a very old part of your brain. They have no interest in explaining themselves to the new kid on the block, the conscious mind, and the conscious mind wouldn't understand anyway. Whatever you felt, that was the emotional trigger that got you out alive. You don't need any more justification than that.

7.3.4: questions

Not everyone survives. There will be an extra helping of disturbing feelings, particularly guilt, if you survived and someone else didn't. It may be compounded if the person who died was someone close or someone you feel you should have protected. It is easy to throw out platitudes: live for the day, it's the will of god, shit happens. If you find comfort in those, go for it.

If you read the chapter The Fight you know a little about luck. Sometimes people die. It happens. Some days it's not you. On one day it will be. (We are all immortal on every day but one. Think that one over.) The question for me is not to look at "why" but to ask, "So what am I going to do with it?" I could be in the cold ground, could be the poor bastard in the body bag, but I'm NOT. What will I do with that gift?

Living in the moment and for the future is almost always healthier than dwelling in the past, agonizing over the "why." The universe does not give a damn about "why." The universe has no need or desire to make sense, certainly not for the benefit of one little human. The entire "why" question is a pathetic little attempt to regain some control ("If I only knew why it happened, why me, why I survived, I might be able to . . .").

It's crucial to know dynamics and the true "why" is usually pretty easy: the guy needed money for drugs, he'd practiced his attack for a long time, he saw that his victim wasn't familiar with the area and probably had some cash, and the victim dropped her guard for a moment.

That's it. Intent, Means, and Opportunity. The search for anything deeper is about ego and amulets. It is about wanting what happened to

191

you to be special and epic in some way; about wanting to believe that all the little vulnerabilities in life (not just crime, but even car accidents and cancer and . . .) don't *usually* apply to you, this was *different*; and even more about finding or inventing something different so that you can use it like a spell or superstition to keep it from happening ever again.

There is a tool that professionals use to deal with the immediate past, particularly failure but anything high-risk. It is supremely effective and simple. It is called an After-Action Debriefing (AAD). It is usually used in groups but you can do it solo. This is another of those tools that will help in every area of your life. There are three steps.

Get as many of the involved people together as you can and as accurately as possible describe what happened. By yourself, with a notebook, play it through in your mind and develop a timeline. Be as detailed and accurate as possible. If you have any little memory tricks like watching things backward or visualization meditation, use those to squeeze out detail. When doing this with a group, I use a dry erase board and start a timeline, letting each person tell what they saw starting with the one who was involved earliest. There will be inconsistencies and disagreements. That is fine. The human memory is fallible.

After the timeline is complete, ask what went well. Here's a big clue: you are breathing so something went well. Lay it out there. This is where you will pick out what some of your most reliable techniques are. This is also where you will find out that you may not be the martial god that you always imagined you would be on the other side of the looking glass, but you're no slouch either with some definite strengths; strengths that have been proven when it counted.

Then you ask: If it happened again, what could we do better? This is not blaming or finger-pointing. There is no room in this process for saying, "I sucked" or "It was all Steve's fault." Nowhere in the process do you ask what anyone did wrong. *What could you do better?* There are some traps to avoid here—it is easy to wish for things or information you didn't have. That is misleading unless you work out a way to have the information next time. ("Wish I'd known he had a knife," is not useful because you didn't know . . . it can however become useful if you then follow it up with, "Maybe I should get some hints on how to tell if a person is packing.") The other trap is trying too hard. Some things, a lot of things, actually, go pretty well. If you look at the scenario and can honestly say, "That ended about as well as it could have," you're done. Trying to improve something that worked is a very human problem that can complicate things to uselessness.

These three steps, applied to anything, will impel constant improvement. It's powerful. Use it.

7.3.5: victim power

Most people have never felt utterly helpless. One of the most devastating aspects of being a victim, especially for men, isn't the injury or the defeat. It is that in the final moments the victim is utterly helpless. The victim, you, may have given it everything you had and it wasn't enough. You weren't enough. It is natural to appeal for help when all is lost and so we have war heroes crying for their mothers as they die and violence survivors whose last clear memory is of begging either their attacker or god for a little more life.

We are monkeys though, and we are the most adaptable animals this planet has ever seen. We will find strength in weakness and power in adversity. And many victims will be seduced by the power they have as victims.

The "victim card" is not just a powerful political ploy, it is a powerful lever in personal relationships as well. Around kind and compassionate people, a former victim can control the entire group just by expressing discomfort. They can say, "I can't go with you, for some reason it reminds me of . . ." and the group will choose another place.

The discomforts are real at first. But your monkey brain, the one that freezes in fights and can't distinguish between mortal danger and embarrassment also understands and craves social power. It will notice that this victim status gives it social power and will try to use it to manage all discomfort.

If you are okay with that it's not my business. Most of humanity for most of human history has sought safety, security, and comfort. It's not my place to tell you that there is something wrong with an effective tactic. I think there are unintended consequences however. I have lost friends who have gone so far down this path that every conversation (even about the weather or sports) was a minefield. At some point it became not just about controlling comfort but about controlling other people, controlling friends. Defensive mechanisms warped into power plays.

It is hard, if not impossible, to cling to the victim power and still be assertive. The problem is that to use the power you have to look and act and think like a victim. In my experience, that reduces every other area of your life. It may be worth it. Only you can decide. In *Meditations on Violence* there is some advice on how to break this cycle. It is not easy and certainly not comfortable.

Victim status also makes a convenient excuse. People tend to be forgiving and understanding if someone who has been through a horrendous event "slips" or "cracks" and, say, beats his wife. That's *not* okay. That is not acceptable on any level. The perpetrator should not

Nature/nurture really doesn't matter. Humans are adaptable and that far outweighs the power of genetic predestination or training. If people know they can't get away with something, they don't try (a cop in the rearview mirror prevents all kinds of bad driving).

If they know that they can get away with something, some will try, depending largely on how responsible they feel to the community.

So nature/nurture in an individual is far secondary to adaptability and utility, but as a philosophy of responsibility it can have profound effects on a society. Humans are adaptable. If you tell them they are and will be held responsible, they will manage their risks and act as if it were true . . . and if you tell them that they had no choice due to genetics or early training, they will act as if that were true as well, and do whatever they damn well please.

There are exceptions, training ingrained by the age of eight or so is very hard to change, but even many vicious Predators become quite civilized in a jail setting where supervision limits their ability to get away with bad behavior.

do it and his peers, support network and the law should not be understanding or forgiving.

If you develop the rage response to being a victim you have to face up to two facts and deal with them.

Fact #1: You wanted to hurt someone you either love or at minimum should care for and protect.

Fact #2: You acted on that desire.

Everything else is bullshit. There is no dark monster lurking inside you. That is just you. There are no uncontrollable urges. Your flashbacks and blackouts are excuses to do what you want and try to avoid responsibility. (If you ever have a blackout and wake up realizing that you've donated bone marrow and given all your money to charity, I'll cut you some slack on this. Every black-out or flashback event I've heard covered actions the person knew to be wrong under normal circumstances.) Maybe that's the third fact you have to face: what you did is you.

You wanted to hurt someone you love? Who hasn't? People you love are sometimes the only people close enough to really hurt us. This desire is not something new. If you think that you never felt anything but warmth and love before your traumatic incident you are not remembering correctly. You are choosing not to remember correctly in order to feel different, special, and privileged now. Yes, privileged. You want the right for you and you alone to act-out without consequences.

If I wish to be charitable I will tell you that you want to be a child again and acting irresponsible is a way of asking for someone else to be responsible and make you feel safe. That's probably true but you aren't a child. You are an adult and being an adult means that you control yourself. That pretty much defines adult. If you blame the incident (or your parents or your genetics or drugs or refined sugar or whatever) for what you do, you are being a child.

And that is the essence of fact #2. You can *feel* any damn thing you want but you are entirely, 100% responsible for whether and how you act on your feelings. "Responsible" means you have no excuses. Truly responsible would mean voluntarily taking the full punishment without complaining. Don't see that much.

7.3.6: friends, society, and alienation

Some say you can never go home. That's not quite true. You step through the looking glass. If all goes well, you come back. You will have changed to some extent and how you see the normal world probably will have changed a lot. How other people see you may well have changed as well. That can be hard.

There are three paths that can lead to an estrangement from society after violence.

If it was a single traumatic event (either you were severely victimized or you took a life) you will be fighting a battle in your head at the same time that your friends and support networks will be trying to figure out what they should do or say. Violence is rare here and now. Just as the victim doesn't have a plan for processing it, it is also new territory for the friends who want to help. The helpers can stumble, make matters worse . . . or more likely they are afraid that they will, and so they withdraw.

Between the victim power and your residual anger, you will be prone to lash out and especially prone to take things wrong. Your monkey mind has powerful incentives for trying to prove to itself that you have control and power (control and power negate fear) and that you are special.

So your friends say, "Are you okay?" And you attack, "Of course I'm not okay!"

Or they try to be encouraging, "You're strong. You'll get over this." And you say or think, "I'll never get over this, you can't possibly understand."

Or the friends say nothing and withdraw. Maybe because they don't know what to say, maybe because they have already tried and you have pushed them away. You find yourself thinking that your friends are afraid or ashamed of you, that you are polluted or have the mark of Cain.

This is an ugly dynamic and has to be hit from two perspectives.

If you are the survivor, cut your friends some slack. Yes, you are hurting and your world has been shattered, but your friends are confused too. Help them. This is one of the magic keys of healing, help

One of the reasons that violence is so traumatic in this day and age is that it has become relatively rare. If you were born and raised when there were no laws or no effective enforcement, when bands of outlaws or competing armies regularly moved through your village taking anything they wanted, violent death and rape might not even seem abnormal to you. The child soldiers of Africa that seem so tragic to our modern minds would not have been an unusual story for much of human history. The props have changed: the spears have become rifles, the chariots have become technicals. The situation is as old as tribal violence.

other people. For the monkey brain, it satisfies the need to feel special and to connect with others. For the more mature part of your brain it proves that you are still valuable and still strong. Maybe not strong in the way you used to believe, but in another way with some hard-won wisdom.

If you are the friend, the two rules are 1) Listen and 2) Don't judge.

Never forget that you are talking to a survivor and despite your fantasies or even experience, there is no guarantee that what you would have done in the same situation would have left you alive. You can listen, you can help them work it out. You can even introduce them to the After-Action Debriefing process to help them work it out. But if your goal is to help them, you don't judge.* You don't have the authority to judge a survivor.

The survivor should be doing most of the talking. Listen. You are helping them process what happened. Let them find their way. Ask them questions, don't try to supply answers.

There is a book, *Aftermath: Violence and the Remaking of a Self*, by Susan J. Brison, that describes her ongoing recovery from a brutal

---

* And if someone is trying to judge or tell you what you did right or wrong they are not trying to help you. They may believe that they are, but what they are really searching for is an amulet that can protect them from whatever happened to you.

attack.* I don't recommend it for survivors. I believe that some of the choices Dr. Brison made in her aftermath were disempowering even as she convinced herself they were great strides in regaining her power. That sounds like a dis, and I apologize. Dr. Brison survived something that very likely would have killed me and there is no guarantee that I could survive even the aftermath (the suicide rate among survivors is high). She has my absolute respect. I don't always agree with people that I respect.

I *do* strongly recommend *Aftermath* for people who work with survivors. It is the best first-person account I have ever read of how people rewrite the story of their identity after a violent attack. Critical information on the process for those who will help with the process.

If the survivor pushes you away, call them on it. Gently point out what they are doing: "I'm trying to be here for you and you're pushing me away. Tell me how I can help." Or, "If that's the wrong thing to say, what's the right thing? What do you want to hear from me?" Or even, "Is there someone else who could make you feel more comfortable than I can?"

The monkey in their brains has been introduced to a brutal dynamic of dominance. It is something we all know is there and pretend isn't. The atavistic power to take what you want, to force your will on others and to kill is a fact of nature. We hang on to our civilized beliefs that we are somehow above that, that it is no longer a danger in our environment. The survivor has just seen that this is not true and there is another world just below the surface of our civilized on where power and violence is life and death. A terrifying world that is potentially as close as the nearest human mind. That world terrified the monkey and the monkey wants to regain its power in that new scary world.

Your job as a friend is to connect with the survivor and with the monkey on the healthy social level. To show that not every relationship has to be a power or predator/prey dynamic. Remind the victim that there are still things like friendship and trust. Don't deny the other world, but put it in perspective. It is real, but trying to use the rules of

* Brison, Susan J.

the looking glass world in the civilized world is just as dysfunctional as trying to stay civilized when attacked.

The single traumatic event can be much harder to recover from than living a violent life. Repeated exposures remove some of the uncertainty of it. In a single event, you mostly learn which of your beliefs was false; in repeated encounters you learn new things to replace the old beliefs. You also get some practice in transitioning between the two worlds. If you practice transitioning with an open mind it can develop an amazing power to adapt to new situations, because you learn how much truth is situational or social. You get better at learning the rules of a new group quickly rather than trying to screen, adapt, or discard your old rules.

You also, over time, get to screen your friends. Some people will not be okay with someone who lives with a fair amount of violence in their lives. Cops make people uncomfortable. Some people, even other cops sometimes, are very uncomfortable with people who are exposed to a fair amount of violence and are comfortable with it.

The thing is, if you have issues or some visible signs of trouble with coping with the violence, peaceful people have an easier time relating to you. They actually come to see you as something slightly broken, damaged. It gives them an excuse to pity you and consequently feel superior to someone that they would otherwise fear.

The fear is real too and it comes from this: if you have successfully dealt with violence for a long time you have developed an ability to flip a switch, to go from happy or smiling or dealing with mundane chores to full-on violence without working yourself up to it (as in the Monkey Dance or looking for hooks). You have an ability to instantly "other" someone based on their behavior. No matter how often you prove that this "othering" is always based on the Threat's behavior, no matter how often you prove your control and judgment, this ability to "other" is terrifying. It brings up a superstitious dread, like a werewolf. A predatory Threat who walks among us and looks like us.

Even Lon Chaney, Jr., always showed some remorse and tried to control his animal side in the old movies. How much scarier is a werewolf who shows no ambivalence, no regret?

People who have successfully immersed in this world screen their friends. They tend to hang with people much like them with similar skills, similar experiences, and similar senses of honor.* Often that means very few friends. Which is fine.

It is often a mistake however. A wise man once told me about the trouble with going into law enforcement as a career, "No matter what any bleeding-heart tells you, 3% of the people in the world are scum. The trouble is, if you spent 80% of your time with that 3%, you start thinking that 80% of the world is scum."

It is critical for people who spend a lot of time with bad people to maintain close ties with good people. Not just with people like themselves but with regular, nice people: teachers and students and cab drivers and nurses and . . . you know, the ones who actually keep society moving.

There are two big hurdles that come with long-term exposure to violence. One is that many people who seek these careers are drawn to it because it seems cool and fun and they are not really fit for it. If it keeps you awake at night, if it makes you want to drink, if you dread going on patrol . . . quit. If you want to do the high-risk stuff, you'd better also have the appetite for training it requires to be safe on the high-risk teams. There are few things worse or more dangerous than the recruit who works his ass off to get on SWAT and then quits working out once he's made the team.

The second is an entirely imaginary belief that you are so special that no one can relate. Dealing with violence can really clarify your values, it can shatter your beliefs, and it can make you give up on the idea of certainty altogether. Transition between enough different kinds of violent and peaceful societies and it becomes apparent that many people know things that aren't true.

---

* Honor is critical. The deepest contempt I have seen from this brotherhood isn't for criminals or corrupt politicians. It is reserved for people like themselves who don't hold themselves to a very high internal standard. Which brings up another thing that scares people, these werewolves can only be restrained by extreme force or an internal standard. External standards are observed as a courtesy, part of the internal code is often to be courteous to the people you are protecting by following their rules.

I'm going to speculate here. You see and hear a lot about alcohol and high-risk professions, about how people turn to alcohol to deal with events. I think that perception is grossly exaggerated. There are some people who drink to forget or dull emotions, more often the ones who thought the job would be cool are in way over their heads and are too egotistical to quit.

The heavy drinkers do it for a different reason, in my opinion. Because they are bored. When you get to the stage that it takes someone shooting at you to get even the slightest trickle of adrenaline, you are bored most of the time. Alcohol, like over-sleeping, becomes just a way to make time pass until something interesting happens.

You transition back to the peaceful world and the office politics that are agonizing for a friend seem silly compared to a knifing. Worrying about your child's grades seems sadly misplaced to a paramedic who has seen a baby decapitated in a car accident. You find yourself listening with glazed eyes as people tell you about their greatest triumphs and trials.

This part really isn't a big deal. I can't speak for everybody but there is a deep comfort and some joy in knowing that most of the world is secure enough where small things can seem like big problems. The real big deal is that you come to believe that people can't handle the truth. That the good people you see around you every day would be in some way damaged or polluted to hear about your world. That's bullshit too, and it is dangerous bullshit. Nice people are tougher than that.

This sense of isolation is something that *we* create and foster. It is imaginary.

Once upon a time, close on the heels of a very dark couple of years, my agency sent me to a "Challenge Course Facilitator" school. This was back when walking tightropes and having very safe but scary-feeling adventures was considered an extraordinary way to build group solidarity. It is, by the way.

I spent a couple of weekends in the woods as the sole thug, a tactical team leader, jail fighter, thug-wrangler, and crazy-calmer in a group of old hippies and fresh college kids most of whom smelled like patchouli and didn't eat meat. It sounds like a recipe for a sit-com or at the very least for violent arguments . . . it didn't happen. The thing about training like this is you have to share and you can't keep it to the surface level.

It was good. I'll tell you the truth, I felt more real than most of them. The things that I shared tended to have a cost and there was a name attached. Where they were dealing with feelings, I tended to be dealing with injuries and damage. ("I don't know if I've ever really been in love" vs. "I wasn't sure if I would lose my sight.")

But we all listened and we all learned. And no one was so fragile that they couldn't hear about some of the violence that shaped me. The isolation that I had been building evaporated very quickly.

No, people who haven't been there won't fully understand. They don't have a frame of reference to really grasp the implications of violence when you describe it, but that's not the important part. The telling and the listening are the important part. Give your friends enough credit. They can and will listen. They'll tell you if they don't want to hear. You don't have to understand in order to care.

There is a third issue that old fighters face—aging. As we grow older our bodies become far less reliable in emergencies. When our identity is attached to surviving emergencies, we tend to get stupid. We pretend that we are still as fast (and heal as quickly) as we used to. I don't have an answer for this one or really any good advice.

The third and rarest type of traumatic change comes from long-term exposure as a continuous victim. As a slave or captive or a continuously abused child (such as Jaycee Dugard, held for eighteen years in California; or Colleen Stan, the subject of the book, *Perfect Victim*) the survivor has a suite of different factors.

The trauma and victimization, of course. There is also the possibility of a complete lack of connection with the normal world. The survivor of a single event is still primarily connected with the normal world. The professional bounces regularly on both side of the looking glass. Someone who has been a captive for extended time may effectively forget that there is a normal world and forget how it works.

Lastly, the captors may have conditioned and taught many behaviors for surviving as a captive, largely growing an entirely new personality in the victim. I am reluctant to guess what the recoveries have been like or what helped or hindered returning to the normal world.

7.4: retaliation

If you are required to use force, after you are safe and have calmed down, you'll have to do a security assessment. Some things aren't over when they are over. Even a low-level Monkey Dance that went to blows can come back to haunt you. Predators sometimes have families and gangs.

The first thing you will have to determine is how much information you have and what information you need. If it was a dust-up at your local watering hole, you already know if Joe Bob has a vindictive streak and keeps a rifle in his truck. Or maybe you don't. Find out. Ask somebody.

If not . . .

Who attacked you?

How soon will he be capable of attacking again? Calling on a cell phone? How much time will it take to marshal his resources for retaliation?

Was he alone—both help and witnesses?

Was this predatory? Monkey Dance?

If predatory, what was the resource? Money? Rape? Reputation?

Was the Threat connected? Gang membership is obvious, but what about local politicians or law enforcement relatives?

If Monkey Dance, what's his reputation? Good loser? Bad loser? Vindictive and will get his own back from ambush?

Social violence usually implies that this information is in the social network and, coincidentally, the social network should be close to where the social violence happened.

If the Threat has criminal ties or history, the police or the prosecutor may be able to supply the information. That information as well will be available on the social network and possibly with fewer hoops.

Most of the time retaliation is not a problem unless you were playing an active part in a "territory in dispute" type of violence. Most Monkey Dancers try to be friends once dominance is established and may not even remember the incident when they sober up. Most Predators are junkies looking for money for drugs and have relatively few friends. Those friends they have are unwilling to take time out of their schedule for vengeance. A drug habit currently can run $800 a day. It takes a lot of time to steal and sell that much.

You will have to estimate from your information how long you will have to be careful (families sometimes have long memories; gangs less so, it must be immediate for the desired effect) and how careful you will have to be (just avoid a certain place? or carry a gun at all times, check under your car before getting in, and move to another city?).

The most common retaliation in this day and age, however, is the threatening letter from an attorney and a civil suit.

AFTERWORD

It's clear that all seven areas are critical. A failure to understand the legalities when you use force can cost you your assets or liberty; an undiscovered glitch can cost you your life in a freeze. Understanding violence can keep bad things from happening; a properly conditioned counter-assault can save your ass. If you don't break the freeze, your fate is in the hands of the bad guy and you will live or die depending on his mood. Once the fight is on, most training will have value, but there may be vulnerabilities as well if the training ignored the natural elements of fighting. And afterwards, when everything should be over and it's happily-ever-after time, you still may face prison or suicide or the slow-motion suicide of trying to self-medicate with drugs and alcohol.

Winning can sometimes seem clear but there are a lot of ways to lose despite an apparent win. If you train to protect yourself and are unaware or misinformed, your training can backfire in ways you may not expect. Aggressive martial arts emphasizing a "finishing blow after the takedown" may actually be conditioning you for excessive force. You might be *practicing* sending yourself to prison.

It is artificial to separate these seven aspects. They affect each other profoundly. How well you integrate the laws of force (Section 1) into your fighting training (Section 6) will have a profound effect on the likelihood of being arrested or successfully sued (Section 7). It all ties together. Finding your internal issues with using force will prevent some of the freezes. Overcoming or training with respect to your glitches will increase your effectiveness in the fight *and* minimize the emotional after-effects.

Understanding the dynamics of violence helps to articulate your decisions in the legal aspects, helps in planning and executing avoidance, and even backtracks and can help you work out some of your glitches.

Everything ties together. The essence of self-defense isn't in a fancy technique or an ability to apply power. It lies in understanding the problem and the context. If you have spent years studying the martial answer to a sudden attack, spend a little time studying the question: What does an attack look like, how does it happen?

Study the context, the where and when of violence. Study the forces, not just physical but social and legal that define modern violence.

If it seems that this book has tremendously complicated your self-defense training, take another look. It has given you more ways to prevail than ever before. Keep your eyes open and be safe.

GLOSSARY

What follows are the terms used in this book that may have specialized or non-standard meanings. Threat, for instance, is capitalized throughout this work when it refers to someone who presents a danger sufficient to potentially justify self-defense.

adrenaline. One of the neuro-hormones that contribute to the Survival Stress Response.

After-Action Debriefing. Process that gathers input from all participants to recreate events and analyze the successes and lessons of the operation.

articulation. The skill at explaining what you did and why.

articulation exercise. A drill for expanding intuition by explaining one's hunches and feelings.

asocial violence. Violence conducted against another species (hunting or slaughtering) or violence performed as if it were against another species.

beliefs. Those things you hold to be true, whether consciously or subconsciously.

blitz. An overwhelming attack.

capability. Something you are physically capable of doing.

capacity. Your emotional ability or limits on exercising your capabilities.

charm. The use of social skills to gain an advantage. Used by predators to get access to victims and to bring them to a place of privacy.

chemical cocktail. Another term for the cascade of stress hormones accompanying the Survival Stress Response.

civil. In a legal matter, suits and disputes between individual citizens and/or corporate entities to determine if harm was done and where responsibility lies.

criminal. In a legal case, Criminal refers to proceedings against an individual conducted by the state to determine if a crime has been committed, if the suspect is guilty of that crime and what the penalty should be.

Drop Step. Suddenly falling into a step, as opposed to shifting weight before moving one's feet. Properly executed a tremendous, untelegraphed speed and power multiplier.

Duty to Act. In some cases an individual will be required by law to engage a Threat. This rarely applies to civilians.

Educational Beat Down (EBD). Social violence conducted to enforce the rules and social norms of a group.

Emotionally Disturbed Person (EDP). Law enforcement term for someone behaving strangely when it is not clear whether the behavior is caused by drugs, mental illness or extreme emotional distress.

escalato. Marc MacYoung's term for increasing ego investment in a conflict. "We've put too much effort into this to back-out now."

ethics. A personal code. An attempt to make morals explicit.

excited delirium. Excited delirium is a condition of unknown etiology. It results in a Threat who is extremely dangerous, often immune to pain, unable to communicate or respond to communication, violent and with a very high temperature.

fight. 1) The application of force between two people attempting to injure or dominate each other. 2) As part of the SSR, one of the in-born responses to fear. 3) That stage of an assault where the victim is able to recover from the freeze sufficiently to defend him or her self.

Fish. A new inmate in a jail or prison.

flight. As part of the SSR, the inborn tendency to run in panic.

Freeze. 1) The state of being frozen. 2) As part of the SSR, the inborn response to go completely still when scared. The most common of the 3F (Fight, Flight, Freeze) responses.

freezing. The act of involuntarily not moving under stress.

glitches. Subconscious hesitations.

Group Monkey Dance (GMD). Social violence conducted to set boundaries/membership or for bonding within a group. When members of a group turn en masse on an outsider or someone who is believed to have betrayed the group.

Intent. Intent is one of the three things that make a legitimate threat. Intents, Means and Opportunity. Intent is the desire and/or intention to harm you or someone else (including self-harm) or to otherwise do something bad.

levels of force. A rough continuum of different categories of technique, ranked by potential for damage: Presence, verbal, touch, pain, damage, deadly.

Means. A Threat's ability to do harm. Size, fists or a weapon can all be means.

Monkey Dance (MD). Human dominance ritual.

morals. A vague sense of right and wrong.

operant conditioning. A system of training to create artificial reflexes.

Opportunity. The Threat's ability to reach his victim with the Means.

posture. A natural tendency to prevent violence by appearing to be big, imposing and/or loud.

preclusion. In a claim of self-defense, preclusion is showing that options other than physical force would not have worked. Other options had been precluded.

Predator. Someone using violence asocially.

Process Predator. A predator whose primary motivation is the violent act itself.

psychotic break. Irrational behavior brought on by severe emotional distress. Incredibly stupid things can seem like good ideas.

Resource Predator. A predator who uses violence to attain another end.

Slipping the Leash. The ability to reject social programming against using force and do what needs to be done as ruthlessly as necessary.

social violence. Violence performed within the species that serves the needs of the group.

Status Seeking Show (SSS). Social violence that deliberately breaks social rules in order to establish a reputation for violence.

stress hormones. A number of hormones and neurotransmitters released into one's system in times of danger including adrenaline (epinephrine), norepinephrine, and endorphins.

structure. Aligning your body so that there is a bone-to-bone connection between your base and where you wish to apply power. Removing anatomical "slop" that wastes power.

submit. Showing a submissive attitude in order to prevent an escalation of social violence.

Survival Stress Response (SSR). The body's complete reaction to intense fear or stress including the cascade of stress hormones and the physical symptoms (tunnel vision, auditory exclusion, loss of fine and complex motor skills, memory distortion, etc.).

Tardive Dyskinesia. A series of symptoms associated with long-term use of anti-psychotic medicines.

Thorazine twitch. See *Tardive Dyskinesia*

Threat. An individual who has the Intents, Means and Opportunity to hurt or kill you, a third party, or in some other way engage in an action that must be stopped.

types of force. To distinguish from levels of force, other distinctions are called types. Knives and firearms are both deadly force and of the same level, but one is a contact weapon, the other ranged and therefore typed by range.

values. A scale of what (objects, people, beliefs) you hold in higher esteem than others.

FURTHER READING

Read as much and as often as you can. This is a big world, filled with many things. In one lifetime (or many) you will never experience all that the world has to offer. So live—live hard. Do things that scare you. Meet people who are mysteries to you. (Where do plumbers learn their trade? How do kindergarten teachers maintain control of a roomful of immature primates? How do South American *campesinos* see the world and how is that different than a Japanese *sarariman*?)

When you can't do those things yourself, read about them. Read the writing of the people who have been and done. You will be amazed.

Be cautious with fiction—the world presented is always cleaner and surer than the world you live in. More importantly most of the authors have never *been and done*, and the worlds become the many-times recycled products of fantasy. It is possibly entertaining. I rarely find it useful.

Be cautious as well with non-fiction. All of the books listed below had something useful. I also disagree with some or all of the authors on points. That's okay. I don't have to be right, nor do the other authors. If someone tries to kill you, *you* need to be right. Question everything. Make up your own mind.

on the human monkey

I used the monkey analogy many, many times. Once you learn to see it, little primate power plays are everywhere. For the most part they are petty, nasty, and unpleasant, but the operant word is "petty." You don't need to play. If there is one thing that can lead humans to a higher, more effective and conscious way of dealing with the universe it will be learning to see when they are acting like monkeys and to choose when it is and isn't appropriate. Both monkeys need to play for the game to work. For greater understanding of this, read:

Conniff, Richard. *The Ape in the Corner Office: How to Make Friends, Win Fights and Work Smarter by Understanding Human Nature.* New York: Three Rivers Press, 2005.

Morris, Desmond. *Manwatching: A Field Guide to Human Behavior.* New York: Harry N Abrams, Inc., 1977.

Morris, Desmond. *The Naked Ape: A Zoologist's Study of the Human Animal.* New York: Dell Publishing, 1999.

on the legal stuff

First, I advise that you get in the habit of reading articles in your local paper and analyzing the force incidents you read there. Most will be officer-involved shootings and most will have a spin. That's good—reading through the spin to winnow facts is a skill. Look for the elements: Intents, Means and Opportunity (Preclusion is not a big thing for officers, they are paid to not run away). How dangerous was the threat? Did an injury result? What would have happened with a lower level of force?

It also becomes excellent practice with your own articulation. A reporter with an agenda is excellent practice—very much like an opposing attorney trying to influence a jury. Learn to pick out facts and to explain why some facts are irrelevant. Here are three suggestions for legal study.

First and foremost READ YOUR STATE STATUTES ON FORCE! Do not leave it to friends or instructors or books like this one. Read them for yourself.

Brown, Carl. *The Law and Martial Arts.* Valencia, California: Black Belt Communications, 1998. (It is probably outdated and didn't have the depth or the focus that I wanted, but it is the only book I know about U.S. law for martial artists.)

Truscott, Ted. *Canadian Law and Self-Defence.* Victoria, BC: Desktop Publishing Ltd., 2004. (Not sure how easy this is to find. If you are based in Canada, read it. Law changes fast, though. Read for principles.)

on dynamics of violence and criminals

Once upon a time I read a book about murderers. The author made the strange assertion that murder is very often a first offense. It didn't square with my experiences. Most importantly, it didn't even square with the examples the author used. Here's my point: everyone has a point of view and a set of beliefs (even me). It is very easy to ignore facts that don't support your beliefs and actively seek sources that support your convictions. We all do this. In every section, but very much here, keep your critical mind on red alert. Especially when the book was written by a criminal. First, books by the good guys.

Allen, Bud and Diana Bosta. *Games Criminals Play.* Roseville, CA: Rae John Publishers, 1981.

Davis, Debra Anne. "Betrayed by the Angel" *Harvard Review* Nov/Dec 2004.

Giduck, John. *Terror at Beslan: A Russian Tragedy with Lessons for American Schools.* Golden, CO: Archangel Group, 2005.

Kane, Lawrence and Kris Wilder. *The Little Black Book of Violence.* Wolfeboro, NH: YMAA Publication Center, 2009.

Klinger, David. *Into the Kill Zone: A Cop's Eye View of Deadly Force.* Hoboken, NJ: Jossey-Bass, 2004.

McGuire, Christine and Carla Norton. *Perfect Victim.* New York, NY: Arbor House, 1988.

Miller, Rory. *Meditations on Violence.* Wolfeboro, NH: YMAA Publication Center, 2008.

Rhodes, Richard. *Why They Kill: The Discoveries of a Maverick Criminologist.* New York: Alfred A. Knopf, Inc., 1999.

Samenow, Stantonf. *Inside the Criminal Mind*. New York: The Crown Publishing Group, 2004.

Strong, Sanford. *Strong on Defense: Survival Rules for You and Your Family's Protection Against Crime*. New York: Atria Books, 1997.
I'm going to suggest a few books written by criminals. There are many more, and all are worth a read. Keep a very, very critical mind. Do not read for how the criminal thinks of himself or how he thinks of his victims. As you read notice how the author is manipulating the reader (you), describing or downplaying heinous actions but with a full dose of justification, presenting himself as the hero or the victim even as he kills.

In some cases it has spread farther, a la George Jackson, a petty armed robber who managed to reinvent himself as a revolutionary and got many people to believe his grandiosity. His narcissistic personality is a contrast to the anti-social personalities of the others . . . but it led to the same place. Using people and killing or getting them killed.

Abbot, Jack. *In the Belly of the Beast*. New York: Vintage Books, 1982.

Jackson, George. *Soledad Brother: The Prison Letters of George Jackson*. Chicago: Lawrence Hill Books, 1994.

Shakur, Sanyika. *Monster: The Autobiography of an L.A. Gang Member*. New York: Grove Press 2004

on people

In the end, all books, fiction or non-fiction, are about people. The author is a person, after all, and so is the reader. What follows are some of the ones that stayed with me or had tools that I found useful. They deal with people, with people under stress, and with communities.

Brison, Susan. *Aftermath: Violence and the Remaking of a Self*. Princeton, NJ: Princeton University Press, 2003.

Brymer, M, A. Jacobs, C. Layne, R. Pynoos, J. Ruzek, A. Steinberg, E. Vernberg, and P. Watson (National Child Traumatic Stress Network and National Center for PTSD). *Psychological First Aid: Field Operations Guide*, 2nd Edition. July, 2006. Available on: www.nctsn.org and www.ncptsd.va.gov.

Gonzales, Laurence. *Deep Survival: Who Lives, Who Dies, and Why*. New York: W.W. Norton and Company, Inc., 2004.

Lisitzky, Gene. *Four Ways of Being Human: An Introduction to Anthropology*. New York: The Viking Press, 1961. Probably extremely outdated, but it was my introduction to the thought that different cultures and different people do, truly, see the world differently. And that many of my ideas of truth were merely beliefs.

Machiavelli, Nicolo. *The Prince*. 1532.

Payne, Ruby. *A Framework for Understanding Poverty*. Highlands, TX: aha! Process. Inc., 2005. *Framework* was recommended to me by a poor kid who had fought his way into the middle class as an adult. The author gets a lot of flack from academics, but those of us who have lived in both the rich and poor worlds have found a lot that resonates.

Ripley, Amanda. *The Unthinkable*. New York: Three Rivers Press, 2009.

Shay, Jonathon: *Achilles in Vietnam: Combat Trauma and the Undoing of Character*. New York: Simon and Schuster, 1995.

Wiesel, Elie. *Night*. New York: Hill and Wang, 1958.

Zupan, Mark and Tim Swanson. *Gimp*. New York: Harper Collins Publishers, 2006. Two glorious insights from Mark Zupan: "But here's the bottom line: At some point, life is going to give you a swift, hard kick to the nuts." And, "Sometimes, the fight is all you get."

other books and resources

I originally tried to suggest books with respect to the chapter headings. That didn't work out. In some areas, such as counter assault, little has been done that is realistic or effective. In others, such as breaking the freeze, there is some academic research but little practical knowledge. Talking about your amygdala is cool at parties, not very useful to think about when you are getting pounded.

On top of that, as has been said before, everything connects—the best books, like *The Professionals Guide to Ending Violence Quickly* would go into almost all of the categories. Other books, outstanding in their fields, such as the U.S. Marine Corps' *Warfighting*, shed light on small aspects of things. Full publication information for these two books appear in the list that follows.

Adams, Ronald J., McTernan, Thomas M. and Remsberg, Charles. *Street Survival: Tactics for Armed Survival*. San Francisco: Calibre Press, 1980.

American Academy of Orthopaedic Surgeons. *Emergency care and Transportation of the Sick and Injured, Ninth Edition*. Sudbury, MA: Jones and Bartlett, 2009.

American National Red Cross. *Advanced First Aid and Emergency Care of the Sick and Injured*. American Red Cross, 1988.

Artwohl, Alexis and Loren W. Christensen. *Deadly Force Encounters*. Boulder, CO: Paladin Press, 1997.

Artwohl, Alexis. "Perceptual and Memory Distortions in Officer-Involved Shootings." *FBI Law Enforcement Bulletin*, October, 2002.

Artwohl, Alexis. "No Recall of Weapons Discharge." *Journal of the Law Enforcement Executive Forum*, May, 2003.

Balor, Paul. *Manual of the Mercenary Soldier*. Boulder, CO: Paladin Press, 1993. Sounds cheesy, but it offered some excellent advice on gathering intelligence in a different culture.

Burrese, Alain. *Hard Won Wisdom from the School of Hard Knocks*. Boulder, CO: Paladin Press, 1996.

Caroline, Nancy. *Emergency Care in the Streets,* 6th ed., rev. and exp. by Nancy Caroline. Sudbury, MA: Jones and Bartlett, 1995.

Carroll, Lewis. *Through the Looking Glass, and What Alice Found There*. MacMillan and Co, Ltd., London: 1872.

De Becker, Gavin. *The Gift of Fear*. Boston: Little, Brown and Company, 1997.

Elgin, Suzette. *The Gentle Art of Verbal Self-Defense*. New York: Barnes and Noble, 1988.
I made a comment in *Meditations on Violence* that you should read books by people who think that their art is the best and no other art is necessary. That attitude may not be true, but someone with that attitude has definitely taken their art to a very high level. Suzette is the representative of talking as the ultimate martial art.

Grossman, Dave. *On Killing: The Psychological Cost of Learning to Kill in War and Society*. Boston: Little Brown and Company, 1995.

Grossman, Dave and Loren Christensen. *On Combat: The Psychology and Physiology of Deadly Conflict in War and in Peace 3rd edition*. Millstadt, Illinois: Warrior Science Publications, 2008

MacYoung, Marc. *A Professional's Guide to Ending Violence Quickly: How Bouncers, Bodyguards and Other Security Professionals Handle Ugly Situations*. Boulder, CO: Paladin Press,1996.

MacYoung, Marc. *Street E and E: Evading, Escaping and Other Ways to Save Your Ass When Things Get Ugly.* Boulder, CO: Paladin Press, 1993.

MacYoung, Marc.: *Violence, Blunders and Fractured Jaws.* Boulder, CO: Paladin Press, 1992.

Office of Justice Programs, U.S. Department of Justice, Bureau of Justice Statistics. *http://bjs.ojp.usdoj.gov*

Peyton Quinn. *Bouncer's Guide to Barroom Brawling.* Boulder, CO: Paladin Press, 1990.

Peyton Quinn. *Real Fighting.* Boulder, CO: Paladin Press, 1996.

Remsberg, Charles. *The Tactical Edge: Surviving High-Risk Patrol.* San Francisco: Calibre Press, 1986.

Siddle, Bruce. *Sharpening the Warrior's Edge: The Psychology and Science of Training.* PPCT Research Publications, 1995.

Thompson, George J. and Jerry B. Jenkins. *Verbal Judo: The Gentle Art of Persuasion.* New York: Harper Collins Publishers, 2004.

The United States Marine Corps. *Warfighting.* New York, NY: Bantam Doubleday Dell Publishing Group,1994.

and, finally, some people

Massad Ayoob (www.ayoob.com). His Lethal Force Institute and Judicious Use of Deadly Force videos have been highly recommended by people I respect. His books and articles are well written and well researched.

Tony Blauer (www.tonyblauer.com). As far as I know, Tony hasn't written a book yet, and I rarely watch videos for training. He is, however, the only person I know who is really working operant-conditioned responses to ambushes. He is doing a lot more as well, but his insights into that crucial quarter-second are invaluable and unduplicated.

Gordon Graham (www.gordongraham.com). Gordon is a former high-ranking police officer who now lectures and consults on risk management . . . and risk management is really what self-defense is all about. The man takes thinking outside the box to a whole new level (such as using a doll—excuse me, an action figure—for back-up). He is funny, smart and drops ideas that can change your entire view of the world casually. He needs to write a book.

INDEX

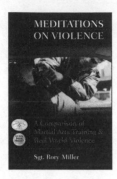

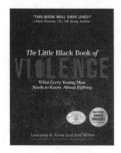

BOOKS FROM YMAA

more products available from ...

YMAA Publication Center, Inc. 楊氏東方文化出版中心

1-800-669-8892 • info@ymaa.com • www.ymaa.com

BOOKS FROM YMAA *(continued)*

TAI CHI WALKING	B23X
TAIJI CHIN NA	B378
TAIJI SWORD—CLASSICAL YANG STYLE	B744
TAIJIQUAN THEORY OF DR. YANG, JWING-MING	B432
TENGU—THE MOUNTAIN GOBLIN	B1231
THE WAY OF KATA	B0584
THE WAY OF KENDO AND KENJITSU	B0029
THE WAY OF SANCHIN KATA	B0845
THE WAY TO BLACK BELT	B0852
TRADITIONAL CHINESE HEALTH SECRETS	B892
TRADITIONAL TAEKWONDO	B0665
WESTERN HERBS FOR MARTIAL ARTISTS	B1972
WILD GOOSE QIGONG	B787
WISDOM'S WAY	B361
XINGYIQUAN, 2ND ED.	B416

DVDS FROM YMAA

ADVANCED PRACTICAL CHIN NA IN-DEPTH	D1224
ANALYSIS OF SHAOLIN CHIN NA	D0231
BAGUAZHANG 1, 2, & 3—EMEI BAGUAZHANG	D0649
CHEN STYLE TAIJIQUAN	D0819
CHIN NA IN-DEPTH COURSES 1—4	D602
CHIN NA IN-DEPTH COURSES 5—8	D610
CHIN NA IN-DEPTH COURSES 9—12	D629
EIGHT SIMPLE QIGONG EXERCISES FOR HEALTH	D0037
ESSENCE OF TAIJI QIGONG	D0215
FIVE ANIMAL SPORTS	D1106
KUNG FU BODY CONDITIONING	D2085
KUNG FU FOR KIDS	D1880
NORTHERN SHAOLIN SWORD —SAN CAI JIAN, KUN WU JIAN, QI MEN JIAN	D1194
QIGONG MASSAGE	D0592
QIGONG FOR LONGEVITY	D2092
SABER FUNDAMENTAL TRAINING	D1088
SANCHIN KATA—TRADITIONAL TRAINING FOR KARATE POWER	D1897
SHAOLIN KUNG FU FUNDAMENTAL TRAINING—COURSES 1 & 2	D0436
SHAOLIN LONG FIST KUNG FU—BASIC SEQUENCES	D661
SHAOLIN LONG FIST KUNG FU—INTERMEDIATE SEQUENCES	D1071
SHAOLIN LONG FIST KUNG FU—ADVANCED SEQUENCES	D2061
SHAOLIN SABER—BASIC SEQUENCES	D0616
SHAOLIN STAFF—BASIC SEQUENCES	D0920
SHAOLIN WHITE CRANE GONG FU BASIC TRAINING—COURSES 1 & 2	D599
SHAOLIN WHITE CRANE GONG FU BASIC TRAINING—COURSES 3 & 4	D0784
SHUAI JIAO—KUNG FU WRESTLING	D1149
SIMPLE QIGONG EXERCISES FOR ARTHRITIS RELIEF	D0890
SIMPLE QIGONG EXERCISES FOR BACK PAIN RELIEF	D0883
SIMPLIFIED TAI CHI CHUAN—24 & 48 POSTURES	D0630
SUNRISE TAI CHI	D0274
SUNSET TAI CHI	D0760
SWORD—FUNDAMENTAL TRAINING	D1095
TAI CHI CONNECTIONS	D0444
TAI CHI ENERGY PATTERNS	D0525
TAI CHI FIGHTING SET	D0509
TAIJI BALL QIGONG—COURSES 1 & 2	D0517
TAIJI BALL QIGONG—COURSES 3 & 4	D0777
TAIJI CHIN NA—COURSES 1, 2, 3, & 4	D0463
TAIJI MARTIAL APPLICATIONS—37 POSTURES	D1057
TAIJI PUSHING HANDS—COURSES 1 & 2	D0495
TAIJI PUSHING HANDS—COURSES 3 & 4	D0681
TAIJI WRESTLING	D1064
TAIJI SABER	D1026
TAIJI & SHAOLIN STAFF—FUNDAMENTAL TRAINING	D0906
TAIJI YIN YANG STICKING HANDS	D1040
TAI CHI CHUAN CLASSICAL YANG STYLE	D645
TAIJI SWORD—CLASSICAL YANG STYLE	D0452
UNDERSTANDING QIGONG 1—WHAT IS QI? • HUMAN QI CIRCULATORY SYSTEM	D069X
UNDERSTANDING QIGONG 2—KEY POINTS • QIGONG BREATHING	D0418
UNDERSTANDING QIGONG 3—EMBRYONIC BREATHING	D0555
UNDERSTANDING QIGONG 4—FOUR SEASONS QIGONG	D0562
UNDERSTANDING QIGONG 5—SMALL CIRCULATION	D0753
UNDERSTANDING QIGONG 6—MARTIAL QIGONG BREATHING	D0913
WHITE CRANE HARD & SOFT QIGONG	D637
WUDANG SWORD	D1903
WUDANG KUNG FU—FUNDAMENTAL TRAINING	D1316
WUDANG TAIJIQUAN	D1217
XINGYIQUAN	D1200
YMAA 25 YEAR ANNIVERSARY DVD	D0708

more products available from...

YMAA Publication Center, Inc. 楊氏東方文化出版中心

1-800-669-8892 • info@ymaa.com • www.ymaa.com